THE SOCIAL IMPACT OF AIDS IN THE U.S.

THE SOCIAL IMPACT OF
AIDS IN THE U.S.

Edited by
Richard A. Berk

Abt Books • Cambridge, Massachusetts

RC
607
.A26
S64
1988
c.1

Library of Congress Cataloging-in-Publication Data

The Social impact of AIDS in the United States.

   Includes bibliographies.
   AIDS (Disease) – Social aspects – United States.
I. Berk, Richard A. (ed.)
RC607.A26S64 1988 362.1'9697'9200973 88-7624
ISBN 0-89011-601-6 (alk. paper)
ISBN 0-89011-602-4 (pbk. : alk. paper)

Copyright © 1988 by Abt Books Inc.

All rights reserved. No part of this publication may be reproduced or transmitted in any form or by any means, electronic or mechanical, including photocopy, recording, or any information storage or retrieval system, without specific permission in writing from the publisher: Abt Books, 146 Mt. Auburn Street, Cambridge, Massachusetts 02138.

Printed in the United States of America

Contents

Introduction The Social Consequences of AIDS: Some Preliminary Observations 1
AIDS and Social Life · The Geographical Distribution of AIDS · The Prospects for a Magic Bullet · Gender, Sex and AIDS · AIDS and the Pornography Industry · AIDS and Hospitals · Educating Physicians · AIDS and the Catholic Church · AIDS and the Press · The Public's Reaction to AIDS · Cross-Cultural Perspectives on AIDS
Richard A. Berk

Chapter 1 Gender, Sexuality and AIDS: Social Responses and Consequences 15
AIDS, Gender and Sexual Behavior Among Heterosexuals · Have Sexual Scripts Changed? · AIDS Prevention Issues Differ for Men and Women · Research Agenda · Men and HIV Infection · Gay Men · Changes in Sexual Practice · Altered Interpersonal Relationships · Confrontations with Death · Male IV Drug Users · Characteristics · The Prospect of an AIDS Death · HIV-Infected Women · Women with AIDS: Neither Male, nor Gay, nor White · Pregnancy and Motherhood · The Female Drug User · Women Living with AIDS · Ethical Issues and Research Questions
Beth E. Schneider

Chapter 2 AIDS and the Pornography Industry: Opportunities for Prevention, and Obstacles 37
The Pornography Industry in Los Angeles · AIDS Research and the Pornography Industry · Estimation of the Prevalence of HIV · Detection of Transmission Dynamics and Estimation of Future HIV Infections · AIDS Intervention Within the Pornography Industry
Paul Abramson

Chapter 3 Looking Back and Forward: Hospital Responses to Epidemics and AIDS 51
Historical Examples · Cholera · Tuberculosis · Venereal Disease · Hospital Responses to AIDS · Finances · Hospital Organization · Discharge Planning · Staff Attitudes and Behavior Responsibility and Refusal to Treat · The Testing Issue · Educational programs · Issues for the Future
Robin Lloyd

· Responsibility and Refusal to Treat · The Testing Issue · Educational programs · Issues for the Future
Robin Lloyd

Chapter 4   AIDS-Related Competencies of Primary-Care Physicians   67
An Overview of the Research · The 1984 Study
Howard E. Freeman, Charles Lewis, Christopher Corey

Chapter 5   AIDS and the Catholic Church   83
The Potential of the Catholic Church · Mobilization of the Los Angeles Archdiocese · The California Catholic Conference · The United States Catholic Church · Catholics Against AIDS: the Praxis · The Latino Question · Linkages · The Effect of AIDS on the Church · Church Doctrine on Homosexuality · Church Doctrine on Birth Control · HIV Testing · Church Membership · Opposition · Cooperation · Appendix A: Latinos and AIDS
Alice Horrigan

Chapter 6   How to Cover a Plague   115
A Note on Methodology · Underplaying an Epidemic · Getting the Story · On the Frontline · Touched by Death · The Politicized Reporter · The Freedom to Be a Reporter · Getting the Facts Straight · How to Cover a Plague · The Future of the AIDS Beat
James Kinsella

Chapter 7   An Attributional Analysis of Changing Reactions to Persons with AIDS   123
Causality, Emotion and Action · Attributional Theory Applied to AIDS · Attributions and Help-Giving · Reactions to AIDS Considered from an Attributional Perspective · The Story of the Ray Children · The Future
Bernard Weiner

Chapter 8   Social Consequences of AIDS: Implications for East Africa and the Eastern United States   133
The Individual · The Couple · The Household, Family, and Clan · Occupational Group · Urban-Rural Populations and Ethnic Groups · More Active and Some Extreme Coping Strategies
Francis Paine Conant

Illustrations

Introduction	AIDS in Los Angeles County by Census Tract 1982–87 *(maps follow page 4)*		
Chapter 4	Table 1. Participation in AIDS Education Programs	70
	Table 2. Test Results after Program	71
	Table 3. Regression and Logit Values for Competence Indicators	72
	Table 4. Primary Care Physicians' AIDS-Related Behavior and Knowledge	74
	Table 4a. Percent of Los Angeles County Adults Asked About Sexual Contacts	75
	Table 5. AIDS Competence Measures and Physician Characteristics	76
	Table 6. Logit Analysis of Predictors of "Overall Competence"	77
	Figure 1. Hypothesized Determinants of AIDS-Related Competence	78
Chapter 7	Table 1. Historical Analysis of Reactions to Persons with AIDS	126
	Table 2. Mean Values for Ten Stigmas	127
	Table 3. Mean Values for Ten Stigmas on Seven Variables Related to Perceived Controllability	129
Chapter 8	Table 1. Paradigms for Size of Groups Affected by AIDS and Strategies for Coping with AIDS	134

Introduction

Richard A. Berk

HISTORIANS HAVE RIGHTLY argued that the course of epidemics is significantly shaped by human institutions and that, in turn, human institutions are altered as an epidemic proceeds. In Brandt's (1987) history of venereal disease in the United States, for example, one finds compelling accounts of the ways in which the transmission of syphilis was affected by the military buildup associated with World War I and by the ways in which military life was organized. In addition, fear of syphilis affected sex education in schools, the treatment of female delinquents, New Deal welfare legislation, tolerance for prostitution, and immigration policy. At a more subtle level, common understandings of cleanliness, health, and morality were influenced. In short, epidemics are inextricably linked to social life and interpersonal behavior.

Aids and Social Life

The current AIDS epidemic is no different (Fineberg, 1988b). The rate of transmission of the retrovirus that causes AIDS, and characteristics of the individuals who become infected, are shaped by a host of collectivities, from formal organizations such as blood banks (Eisenstaedt and Getzen, 1988), massage parlors and public baths (Richwald et al., 1988) to loose collections of individuals in "marriage markets" (Baldwin and Baldwin, 1988), and "shooting galleries" (Ginzberg, 1986; Booth, 1988). Likewise, to the degree that significant and effective prevention programs are to be mounted, schools (Kass, 1987), prisons (Vaid, 1987), business establishments (Rothstein, 1987), military bases (Rivera, 1987), and other institutions necessarily will be involved.

But, just as social entities influence the course of the AIDS epidemic, creating settings for both transmission and prevention, social entities are themselves affected by the epidemic (Berk, 1987). In numerous locales, for example, the delivery of medical services for many different kinds of illnesses is in jeopardy because resources are being diverted to the growing number of individuals with AIDS. Local health departments, especially in some major metropolitan areas, will also be hard hit (Rowe and Ryan, 1988). A recent study by the firm of Peat Marwick Main & Co. (1988),[1] for instance, projects for the 1990s a dramatic shortfall in funding for the Los Angeles County Department of Public Health.

For the nation as a whole, Scitovsky and Race (1987) estimate that between 1987 and 1991, the direct medical expenses associated with AIDS will reach a total of about $8.5 billion. Thus, by 1991 "only the costs of automobile accidents will exceed the medical care costs of AIDS . . ." (Scitovsky and Rice, 1987: 65). Bloom and Carliner (1988) estimate somewhat higher costs, and stress that much of the financial burden will be carried by a few urban areas. Clearly, the health care delivery systems will be sorely taxed in those sites. As national programs such as Medicaid struggle under the strain, the ripples will be felt throughout the country (Inglehard, 1987; Sisk, 1987; Pascal, 1987).

Other sectors of the society will confront similar consequences, perhaps with a slightly longer time horizon. Prisons, already overcrowded and often under court order, may now need to fundamentally change housing practices. Indeed, with the New York State prison system reporting about fifteen percent infection rates among prisoners from New York City (*Criminal Justice Newsletter*, 4/15/88: 1–2), about half of the states now segregate prison inmates who have AIDS, and several states have recently begun testing their inmate populations for seropositivity (Hammett, 1986; Kleinman, 1986). There are also a number of legislative proposals with important general implications for correctional activities. For example, California Senate Bill 1913 was recently introduced into the legislature and included the following provisions:

1. provides procedures whereby a corrections or CYA officer, CHP, police or sheriff's deputy can obtain testing of an inmate who may be an AIDS carrier, if the officer has come into contact with a person's body fluids. . .

2. provides the same procedure for inmates and persons in custody. . .

3. provides for hearings, appeals and confidentiality with penalties. . .

4. requires notification of parole or probation officer if parolee has AIDS when the parolee or probationer is released from prison or custody. . .

---

[1] The study done by Peat Marwick Main & Co. was commissioned and funded by the Los Angeles County Department of Public Health.

5. permits AIDS testing of groups of inmates if a medical officer and hearing panel concludes that a medical emergency exists...

6. requires correctional institutions to provide education, safety, precautions and notification to staff and inmates of AIDS dangers...

7. permits parole and probation officers to notify a spouse if parolee has AIDS...

8. permits notifying police officers in the case that a violent confrontation with a parolee is imminent...

The courts also are facing serious challenges. *U.S. News and World Report* (January 12, 1987: page 62) asserts that "the disease has already wrought a legal tangle of near-unprecedented proportions for Americans...[because] thousands of AIDS victims have been denied housing, schooling, dental treatment, insurance, and jobs." As legal scholar Bernard M. Dickens notes (1988: 580),

> The impact of the acquired immunodeficiency syndrome (AIDS) on human interactions mediated by law has been felt at all levels of society. Early questions about legal protections against the spread of infection are now balanced by questions about the rights of those infected with the human immunodeficiency virus (HIV) and about confidentiality and non-discrimination. The recognition of such AIDS patients as children infected prenatally or recipients of contaminated blood in transfusions has mitigated an early response within the general population that those infected were culpable and undeserving of legal rights (1988:580).

Insurance companies are currently facing how best to spread their AIDS-related financial risks in an environment full of legal and ethical constraints (Hammond and Shapiro, 1986; Faden and Kass, 1988). Some claim that under current reimbursement policies, they are facing financial ruin. And the entire U.S. economy may soon be forced to respond to the AIDS threat. The March 3, 1987 issue of *Business Week* reports estimates that AIDS will cost the country more than $55 billion by 1991 in lost productivity, illness, and premature death. More recently, Scitovsky and Rice (1967) put the figure at $66 billion. Bloom and Carliner (1988) are less pessimistic, but all such figures typically exclude a number of important indirect costs, such as those associated with mounting large-scale education programs, institutional responses to the epidemic, and the increasing use of selective, mandatory testing.

The list of institutions affected could easily be expanded to encompass virtually every organization and sector, including school systems (Kass, 1987), employers (Leonard, 1987; Chelimsky, 1988), and the military (Rivera, 1987). A focus on institutions and organizations must not be allowed to obscure, however, equally important processes operating on social relations within the society at large.

In particular, there are social consequences for groups who are recognized as "high-risk." Gays are obviously one example. Dramatic modifications have occurred in the past decade or so in the community standing of Gays, and gay-rights groups have successfully reduced the extent to which there is overt social and employment discrimination. Yet hostility continues to characterize relationships with many people in the larger community, and public reactions to AIDS have the potential of not only setting back recent gains for Gays, but provoking serious restrictions on their employment opportunities, residential choice, and participation in political, voluntary, and other community activities (Parmet, 1986).

Gays are hardly the only stigmatized high-risk group. AIDS testing in the military, coupled with other indicators, reveals that ethnic minorities will be especially hard hit (Roger and Williams, 1987; Curran et al., 1988). Among young men entering the army, the seropositive rate is about four times higher for Blacks than Whites (with Hispanics in between). Differential rates of intravenous drug use by ethnicity further underscore that social characteristics (poverty, age, etc.), as well as sexual preference, are linked to risk. Thus, any efforts to single out high-risk groups for special concern, even if the concern is benign, immediately become entangled in the persistent community problems of social inequality and discrimination. Indeed, some have directly linked AIDS to the many problems of the "underclass." As Mincy and Hendrickson observe (1988:7),

> In sum, even without the capacity to answer precisely whether areas with higher incidence of AIDS are also underclass areas, piecing together indirect evidence on geographic correlation, demographic distribution, and behavioral correlates of AIDS cases and corresponding information about the underclass area population strongly suggests that high levels of AIDS are found in underclass areas (1988:7).

To summarize, AIDS has direct and indirect impacts on individuals, *and* individual behavior has direct and indirect impacts on AIDS. These reciprocal relationships unfold within the larger context of human collectivities and communities, each of which may leave their own distinct mark on what unfolds. The role of AIDS in the military, for example, may be very different from the role of AIDS in schools or prisons. These would seem to be substantive issues central to academic social science. Perhaps more important, the ongoing relationships between AIDS and social phenomena raise questions of public policy that will no doubt be saliently represented on the political agenda for years to come.

The Geographical Distribution of AIDS

The relationships between AIDS and social phenomena will depend fundamentally upon the geographical distribution of the disease. It is readily apparent that AIDS is disproportionately concentrated in a few major metropolitan areas, especially New York, San Francisco and, at a somewhat lower level, Los Angeles (e.g., Allen and Curran,1988). In Los Angeles County, for example, there were, in the spring of 1988, an estimated 4500 diagnosed cases of AIDS (Peat Marwick Main & Co. 1988). Blacks accounted for fourteen percent of the cases, Hispanics for fifteen percent, and Whites for sixty-nine percent. The vast majority (eighty-two percent) were homosexual and bisexual men, who were not IV drug users. IV drug users represented only about eleven percent of all diagnosed cases. The number of ARC (AIDS Related Complex) cases was estimated to be approximately 3000.

AIDS in Los Angeles County by Census Tract

1982–1987

*(Spatial data courtesy of the
Los Angeles Department of Public Health)*

Aids in LA County by Census Tract 1982

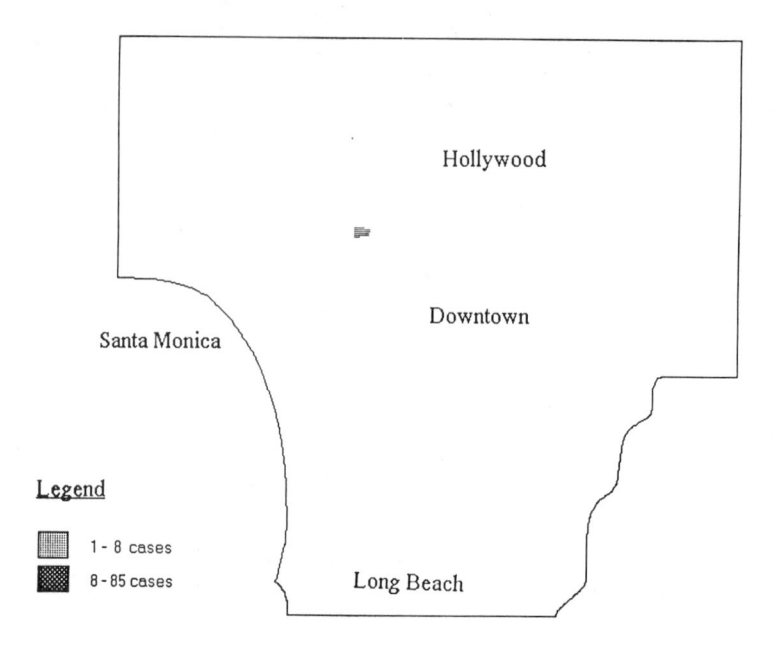

Legend

- 1 - 8 cases
- 8 - 85 cases

Aids in LA County by Census Tract 1983

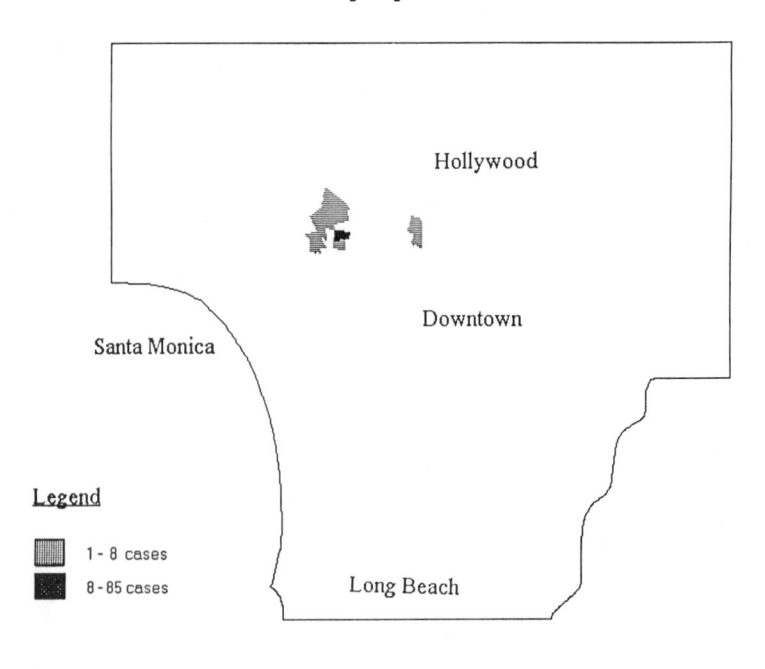

Legend

- 1 - 8 cases
- 8 - 85 cases

Aids in LA County by Census Tract 1984

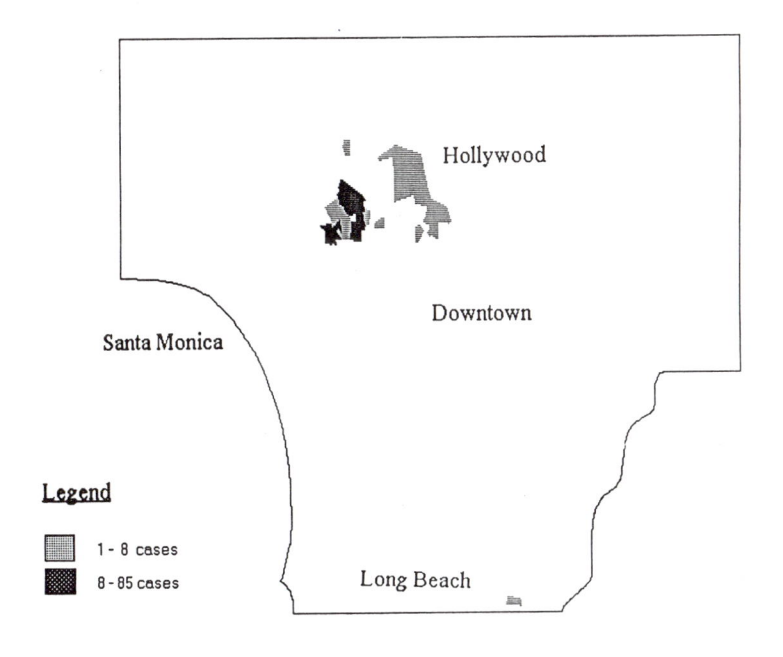

Hollywood

Downtown

Santa Monica

Long Beach

Legend
- 1 - 8 cases
- 8 - 85 cases

Aids in LA County by Census Tract 1985

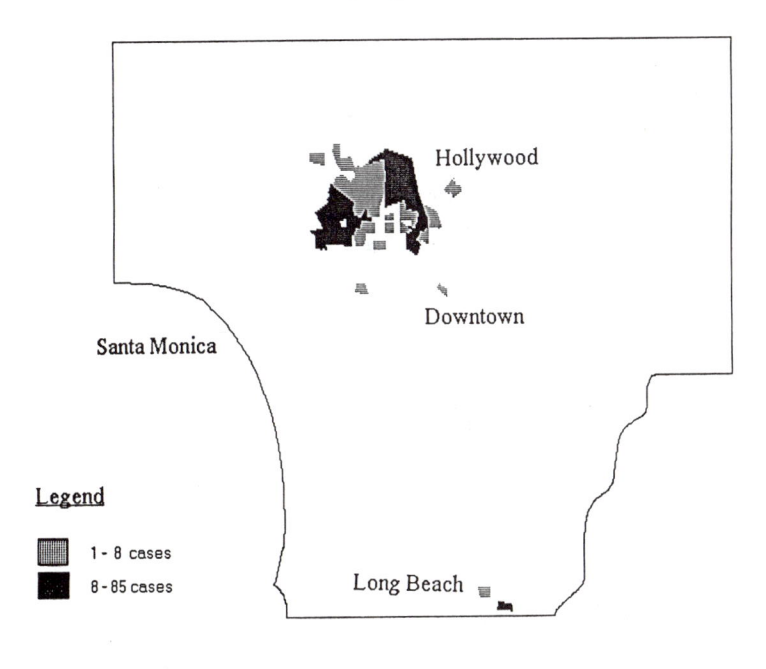

Hollywood

Downtown

Santa Monica

Long Beach

Legend
- 1 - 8 cases
- 8 - 85 cases

Aids in LA County by Census Tract 1986

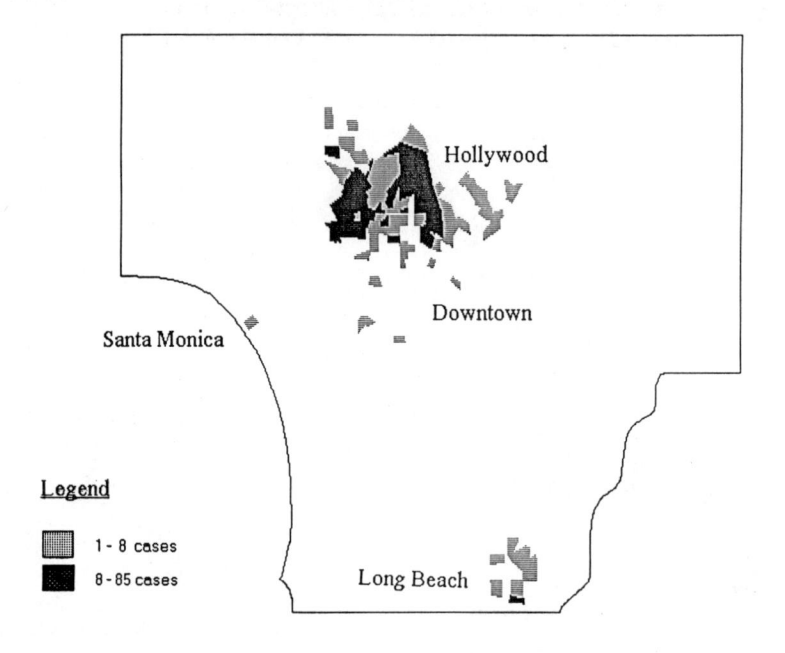

Legend
- 1 - 8 cases
- 8 - 85 cases

Aids in LA County by Census Tract 1987

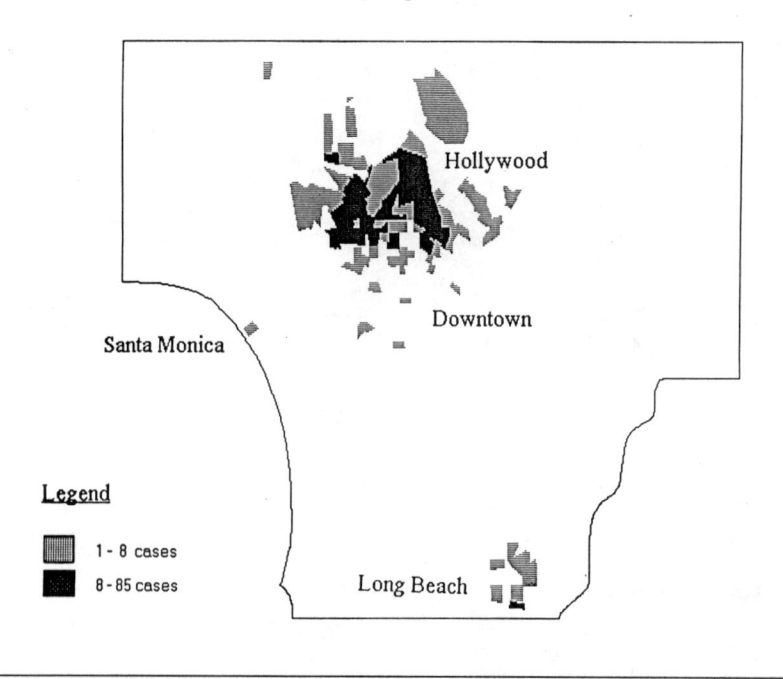

Legend
- 1 - 8 cases
- 8 - 85 cases

Making projections from such modest numbers is a tricky business. Nevertheless, the Peat Marwick Main study projects that by 1991, there will be between 19,000 and 44,000 cases of AIDS in Los Angeles County as a whole. For 1991, this translates into an estimated number of individuals infected with HIV of between 180,00 and 340,000! Even if these figures are on the high side, they demonstrate that the major impact of AIDS has yet to be felt.

One can get a sense of the future by examining graphs 1-6. On each graph is shown for Los Angeles County the number of AIDS cases by census tract. Six years are represented: 1982 through 1987. Clearly, the Hollywood area has had the highest concentration of AIDS cases, but the numbers of cases and their geographical dispersion have been increasing dramatically. By 1987, a significant number of AIDS cases can be found in South Central Los Angeles, Santa Monica, and Long Beach.

In short, despite widespread concern about AIDS among certain public officials and organized groups, and about a true epidemic among Los Angeles Gays, much of the County is in a "pre-test" phase. As the epidemic grows and spreads, the filtering down of effects on social phenomena has only just begun; the worst of the epidemic lies ahead. The bulk of the social consequences has yet to materialize. It cannot be overemphasized that in the next three years, the number of AIDS cases is expected to increase by at least *a factor of five.*

There are perhaps three lessons that may be learned from the Los Angeles experience. First, figures for the country as a whole obscure the seriousness of the AIDS epidemic for certain locales. Second, many of these hard-hit areas are important centers of economic and social activity; they are points of high leverage for the wellbeing of society. If social and economic life in New York, San Francisco and Los Angeles are dramatically affected by AIDS, the ripple effects across the nation will be large and widespread. Third, with the possible exception of San Francisco, the most dramatic effects of the epidemic are yet to be felt. Current experience no doubt seriously understates the difficulties that lie ahead.

Prospects for a Magic Bullet

Up to this point, I have argued that AIDS is already having important social consequences, that these are to date concentrated in a few major metropolitan areas, and that our society has had only a taste of things to come. But some may argue that medical science will soon develop means to at least halt the growth of the epidemic.

Unfortunately, there is widespread consensus that no "technical" fix for AIDS is on the horizon. The prospects for a general vaccine are grim in the medium term (Barnes, 1988; Mathews and Bolognesi, 1988), and the prospects are only slightly better for treatments which significantly reduce the impact of the virus on the immune system (Hirsch and Kaplan, 1987; Yarchoan et al., 1988). Consequently, it is very unlikely that medical developments will significantly alter current predictions for the early 1990s.

Perhaps one might also hope that various kinds of educational efforts will do the job that medical science cannot. Here too, unfortunately, there is little comfort to be found. As Finebery observes:

> For the most part, those who will develop AIDS in the next 5 years have already been infected with HIV-1. Even a spectacularly successful AIDS education program could not alter the course of the epidemic in

the near term. The best that prevention of virus transmission can achieve is a reduction in cases of clinical disease in the intermediate and long terms (1988:595).

And what are the chances of ever developing a "spectacularly successful" educational program? Fineberg lists five major obstacles (1988: 593–594):

1. Sexual behavior and drug use derive from strong biological impulses that are hard to resist.

2. There is still widespread controversy about the content of AIDS education programs.

3. The precise risks from AIDS faced by most Americans remain somewhat unclear.

4. Public officials have often given unclear, or even contradictory, messages about AIDS.

5. Dramatic and sustained changes in behavior will be necessary to affect the course of the epidemic.

To these I would add at least four more:

1. Some key target populations (IV drug users, minorities, and sexually active teenagers) are highly suspicious of information provided by the larger society.

2. Even if there were agreement on what information to provide, there is little scientific information about how best to *deliver* it.

3. Only recently has attention been directed to how educational programs might vary depending on the target population and the particular behavior to be altered.

4. Very little attention has been directed toward rigorously evaluating the effectiveness of AIDS education programs, so there will be little credible information on which programs to expand and which to terminate.

In the face of these difficulties, it should not be surprising that the initial returns on educational efforts are not especially promising. In addition to outright failures (Baldwin and Baldwin, 1988; Kegeles et al., 1988), Fineberg observes (1988: 594–595) that the few successes to date either have been very modest or are arguably not the result of some educational program. For example, although it is clear that a very large number of Gays in San Francisco have dramatically altered their sexual behavior, one cannot determine whether the changes resulted from conscious education efforts or their painful experience of seeing so many in the community succumb. Moreover, "The reduction of

HIV-1 transmission found in recent years in the homosexual population of San Francisco brings scant comfort when half or more are already infected" (Fineberg, 1988: 595).

Despite these realities, major investments must be made in both technical and educational fixes; they hold the hope for the future. There is little hope, however, that either will substantially affect the course of the epidemic until the 1990s. In the meantime, we must learn to cope with the social consequences of AIDS.

The Chapters to Follow

The AIDS epidemic has raised a number of concerns touching on a large number of social phenomena, approached from a wide variety of perspectives. Most of these concerns, in addition, translate into questions that researchers have only begun to address. Consequently, the chapters included in this book, while focusing on the social consequences of AIDS, reflect enormous heterogeneity, and offer research agendas more than research results. In short, the contents of this book are but a very tentative beginning.

Gender, Sex and AIDS

The first chapter, written by sociologist Beth E. Schneider, addresses how AIDS has affected gender relations and sexual behavior. The perspective is dynamic; individuals "do" gender and individuals "do" sexuality. That is, the focus is on process, and the ways in which process affects and is affected by more stable features of the society. The introduction of AIDS into ongoing interpersonal relations is not seen as some pure exogenous intervention, but as a force whose social meaning and import changes as it affects its interactional environment.

For example, Schneider argues that the ways in which couples talk about AIDS depend on an existing menu of slang and euphemisms, which by and large represent the consciousness of men. At the same time, the romantic overlay that many women introduce may represent a wholly different set of concerns. In both instances, there is a significant disjuncture between the need for "straight talk" about sex and the conceptual and linguistic apparatus available. Yet, for those couples who manage some approximation of straight talk, "sexual scripts" may be rewritten.

AIDS and the Pornography Industry

Psychologist Paul Abramson focuses in the second chapter on the pornography industry. In addition to providing a fascinating account of how the industry is organized, he describes concerns about AIDS that have been growing among the various individuals who are involved: actors and actresses, producers, agents, directors, and distributors. He also notes that despite ample opportunities for transmission of AIDS, few of the actors or actresses seem to have contracted AIDS. Perhaps this reflects nothing more than the lag between infection and symptoms, or perhaps the particular practices actually photographed are less risky than one might suspect. Regardless, despite the actions of a few prominent actors and actresses, there is no evidence to date that AIDS has dramatically affected the sexual activities typically filmed.

Against this background, Abramson provides an rich research agenda coupled to an important set of public policy questions. For example, should the pornography industry be given the same scrutiny as bath houses? Would mandatory testing make sense? Might not pornographic films be used to educate about safer sex? In retrospect, it is surprising that the pornography industry has received so little attention in public discussions about AIDS.

AIDS and Hospitals

Studies of the economic impact of AIDS are now routinely available, especially those addressing the economic impact on health care systems. It is surprising, though, that there has been virtually no careful study of how AIDS interacts with and affects the social organization of hospitals; there is more to institutions than dollars.

In the third chapter, therefore, sociologist Robin Lloyd uses the historical backdrop of some past epidemics to explore the fit between the needs of AIDS patients and the services that hospitals are organized to provide. In many ways the fit is poor. For example, hospitals are far better equipped to handle acute medical problems than they are to provide long-term care. One consequence of the organizational focus on acute care is that treatments are typically imposed on patients. Yet, for people with AIDS, a more collaborative approach seems required; patients might well benefit from participating more fully in decisions about the care they need and about how it should be provided. Another consequence is that the needs of people with AIDS for a wide variety of medical and support services is typically overlooked. That is, in contrast to usual practice, it seems important to construct a *package* of medical and social services, whose contents can be altered as the disease progresses. Lloyd argues, however, that in some hospitals at least, AIDS is forcing a re-examination of conventional practice and, in a few instances, fundamental organizational change has taken place. Perhaps, this re-examination will affect hospital organization more generally.

Educating Physicians

The current concern about public education on AIDS seems to take for granted the expertise of the medical community. Perhaps it is simply assumed that medical practitioners can be brought quickly up to speed, since keeping current with medical advances in part defines good medical care. In Chapter 4, sociologists Howard Freeman and Christopher Corey, and physician Charles Lewis, explore how primary-care physicians — general practitioners, internists, and family medicine specialists — are responding to the AIDS epidemic. Primary-care physicians are an essential part of the medical response to AIDS since they are in a position to help with prevention, to provide early and accurate diagnoses, and to follow-up on treatment programs.

Summarizing the results of two unusually well-designed studies, Freeman and his colleagues conclude that a large proportion of primary-care physicians are not yet able to competently discharge their duties in the case of AIDS patients. Moreover, a specially designed educational program for primary-care physicians had almost no impact. In short, neither the day-to-day experiences associated with medical practice nor the usual sorts of educational efforts are likely to change quickly the practices of primary-care physicians. Or in the authors' own words, "To put it bluntly, the secular changes in knowledge that are occurring among primary-care physicians probably are not much different from those taking place among regular readers of *Time* or *Newsweek*." In an important sense, AIDS is having *no* impact. At the same time, however, the authors offer a number of suggestions about how more intrusive educational efforts might be successful.

AIDS and the Catholic Church

The Catholic Church is clearly a powerful institution. The Church preaches on a regular basis to an audience of millions and more widely is able to reach individuals who at least grant the Church some moral authority. In addition, the Church is a mighty political organization that is able to affect the views and actions of other institutional actors. It is hard to imagine, for example, that an AIDS education program could be launched in public schools over the Church's opposition.

Sociologist Alice Horrigan examines in Chapter 5 how the Catholic Church in the Archdiocese of Los Angeles has reacted to the AIDS epidemic, especially with respect to its Latino parishioners. She finds surprising heterogeneity within the Church: differences between public statements and private actions, differences between the pronouncements of Church leaders and the day-to-day activities of parish priests, and a movement among some clerics toward a fundamental reassessment of the nature of homosexuality and human sexuality more generally.

For example, the Church has long held that having a homosexual preference is by itself not sinful. Acting on that preference, however, is prohibited. Some critics have argued that the juxtaposition of these two views is at least insensitive (some use the word "sadistic"), especially when the sexual act is part of a longstanding monogamous relationship. As a growing number of parish priests help care for people with AIDS, the critics' position is getting a more serious hearing. AIDS has also stimulated considerable discussion about sex education, birth control, and heterosexual behavior.

AIDS and the Press

In Chapter 6, James Kinsella, editor of the editorial pages of the Los Angeles *Herald Examiner*, considers how AIDS has been characterized by the media and how in turn AIDS may affect media practices in the future. Some readers may be surprised to learn about the degree to which extrinsic factors determine what is reported and the manner in which the story is written. A newsworthy event must be "good copy," the nature of which depends on judgment calls subject to a host of formally irrelevant criteria. For example, the perceived importance of a story may depend in part on the idiosyncratic personal experiences of a particular reporter, which stimulate sensitivities that might otherwise be unreachable; in some sense, the reporter has to care.

Perhaps more important over the long run is how media reporting on AIDS is being shaped by the very process of covering it. For example, the level of medical sophistication has increased enormously and graphic language about sexual behavior is now commonly used. More broadly, there is a growing understanding about the uncertainty of all scientific findings and an appreciation that science is an evolving collective process, not a fixed body of procedures.

The Public's Reaction to AIDS

While it is clear that AIDS triggers within the public a complex set of highly charged emotions, it is difficult to understand the dynamics. Why, for example, does there seem to be sympathy for hemophiliacs with AIDS and hostility for homosexuals with AIDS? Is this simply a reflection of sentiments about homosexuals? And, what may help account for the growing public support for AIDS research and the medical care for persons with AIDS? Is this simply a reflection of concerns about the spread of AIDS among heterosexuals?

In Chapter 7, psychologist Bernard Weiner applies attribution theory to help explain evolving public attitudes about AIDS. Summarizing research findings from several experimental studies, he links perceptions of hostility to beliefs that, for IV drug users and homosexuals, the transmission of AIDS may in principle be prevented. Moreover, IV drug users and homosexuals have the capacity to prevent transmission, and apparently choose not to act. That is, the public's lack of sympathy for people with AIDS may have more to do with the attribution of responsibility than with moral abhorrence for homosexual behavior or IV drug use.

Cross-Cultural Perspectives on AIDS

Social scientists have long been torn between two distinct views of social phenomena. On the one hand, a social *science* requires continuities across human behavior or generalization becomes impossible. On the other hand, there is a general acknowledgment that all human behavior has unique content.

In Chapter 8, anthropologist Francis Conant forces AIDS researchers to confront this dilemma by speculating about the social consequences of AIDS for the Eastern United States and social consequences of AIDS for East Africa. He distinguishes between two dimensions of responses to AIDS, one based on the size of the affected group and one based on various coping strategies. With respect to size, for example, he contrasts social consequences for the household to social consequences for a regional population. With respect to coping strategies, he defines three kinds of activities: passive, active, and violent. Denial is an illustration of a passive strategy, scapegoating is an illustration of an active strategy, and suicide is an example of a violent strategy. Crossing his two dimensions, Conant then speculates about a variety of scenarios. Conant's chapter is important not just because it greatly broadens the perspective one might apply to the social consequences of AIDS, but because it introduces cross-national content that is, unfortunately, largely missing in the other chapters.

Conclusions

The justification for this volume rests in part on the assumption that significant public resources will be invested over the next several years to manage the social consequences of AIDS. An intelligent marshalling of those resources requires that an effort be made to anticipate what the social consequences of AIDS will be.

The essays collected here are meant to highlight various aspects of social life that may be affected by AIDS. Most of the chapters are essentially research agendas, and clearly many important topics are not represented. If this book helps to stimulate future research with wider coverage, drawing heavily on new data sets and speaking consistently to policy concerns, it will have been an enormous success.

References

1. Baldwin, John D. and Janice I. Baldwin. 1988. "Factors Affecting AIDS-related Sexual Risk-Taking Behavior among College Students." 1988. *The Journal of Sex Research* 25:2 181–196.

2. Barnes, Deborah, 1988. "Obstacles to an AIDS Vaccine." *Science* 240 719–721.

3. Berk, Richard A. 1987. "Anticipating the Social Consequences of AIDS: A Position Paper." *The American Sociologist* 18:3 3–33.

4. ——————, (ed.) 1988. *The Social Impact of AIDS in th U.S..* Cambridge, Mass.: Abt Books.

5. Bloom, David E. and Geoffrey Carliner. 1988. "The Economic Impact of AIDS in the United States." *Science* 239:5 604–610.

6. Booth, William. 1988. "AIDS and Drug Abuse: No Quick Fix." *Science* 239: 717–719.

7. Brandt, Allan M. 1987. *No Magic Bullet: A Social History of Venereal Disease in the United States since 1880* (revised edition). New York: Oxford Press.

8. —————— 1988b. "AIDS in Historical Perspective: Four Lessons from the History of Sexually Transmitted Diseases." *American Journal of Public Health* 78:4 367–371.

9. Carmichael, Ann G. 1986. *Plague and the Poor in Renaissance Florence.* Cambridge: Cambridge University Press.

10. Chelimsky, Eleanor. 1988. "GAO's Approach to AIDS in the Workplace." *The GAO Journal* 1:Spring 31–38.

11. Curran, J.W., H.W. Jaffe, A. M. Hardy, W.M. Morgan, R.M. Selik, T.J. Dondero. 1988. "Epidemiology of HIV Infection and AIDS in the United States." *Science* 239:5 610–616.

12. Cutler, John C. and R. C. Arnold. 1988. "Venereal Disease Control by Health Departments in the Past: Lessons for the Present." *American Journal of Public Health* 78:4 372–380.

13. Dickens, Bernard M. 1988. "Legal Rights and Duties in the AIDS Epidemic." *Science* 239:5 580–585.

14. Eisenstaedt, Richard S. and Thomas E. Getzen. 1988. "Screening Blood Donors for Human Immunodeficiency Virus Antibody: Cost-Benefit Analysis." *American Journal of Public Health* 78:4 450–455.

15. Fineberg, Harvey V. 1988. "Education to Prevent AIDS: Prospects and Obstacles." *Science* 239:5 592–596.

16. —————— 1988b. "The Social Dimensions of AIDS." *Scientific American,* 256:4 128–135.

17. Ginzberg, Harold M. 1986. "Intravenous Drug Abusers and HIV Infection: A Consequence of Their Actions." *Law, Medicine & Health Care* 14:4–5 268–272.

Introduction

18. Hammett, Theodore, M. 1986. *AIDS in Correctional Facilities: Issues and Options.* Washington, D.C.: U.S. Department of Justice, National Institute of Justice.
19. Hammond, J.D. and A.F. Shapiro. 1986. "AIDS and the Limits of Insurability." *The Milbank Quarterly* 64:1 143–167.
20. Hirsch, Martin S., and Jaon C. Kaplan. 1987. "Antiviral Therapy." *Scientific American* 256:2 76–85.
21. Inglehard, J.K. 1987. "Financing the Struggle Against AIDS." *New England Journal of Medicine* 317:3 180–184.
22. Kegles, Susan M., Nancy E. Adler, and Charles E. Irwin Jr. 1988 "Sexually Active Adolescents and Condoms: Changes Over one Year in Knowledge, Attitudes and Use." *American Journal of Public Health,* 78: 460–462.
23. Faden, Ruth R. and Nancy C. Kass. 1988 "Health Insurance and AIDS: The Status of State Regulatory Activity." *American Journal of Public Health* 74:4 437–439.
24. Fischer, Craig (ed). 1987. *Criminal Justice Newsletter* 19:8 1-3, New York: Pace Publications.
25. Kass, Frederic C. 1987. "Schoolchildren with AIDS." In *AIDS and the Law,* edited by Harlon L. Dalton, Scott Burns and the Yale AIDS Law Project. New Haven: Yale University Press.
26. Kleinman, Mark. 1986. "The AIDS Epidemic and the Criminal Justice System." Program in Criminal Justice Policy and Management, John F. Kennedy School of Government, Harvard University.
27. Kreiger, Nancy and Joyce C. Lashof. 1988 "AIDS, Policy Analysis, and the Electorate: The Role of Schools of Public Health." *American Journal of Public Health* 78:4 411–417.
28. Lang W. Robert, Frederick R. Snyder, David Losovsky, Vivek Kaisha, Mary Kaczaniuk, Jerome Jaffe, and the ARC Epidemiology Collaborating Group. 1988. "aphic Distribution of Human Immunodeficiency Virus Markers in Parenteral Drug Abusers." *American Journal of Public Health,* 78:4 443–446.
29. Leonard, Arthur S. 1987. In *AIDS and the Law,* edited by Harlon L. Dalton, Scott Burns and the Yale AIDS Law Project. New Haven: Yale University Press.
30. Mathews, Thomas T. and Dani P. Bolognesi, 1988. "AIDS Vaccines." *Scientific American,* 259:4 120–127.
31. McNeil, William H. 1976. *Plagues and People.* New York: Anchor Press.
32. Mincy, Ronald B. and Susen E. Hendrickson. 1988. "AIDS and the Underclass: Statement Before the Presidential Commission on the Human Immunodeficiency Virus Epidemic." Washington, D.C.: The Urban Institute.
33. Parmet, Wendy E. 1986. "AIDS and the Limits of Discrimination Law." *Law, Medicine & Health Care* 15:1–2 61–72.
34. Pascal, A. 1987. "The Costs of Treating AIDS under Medicaid: 1986-1991." Washington: D.C.: U.S. Department of Health and Human Services.
35. Peat Marwick Main & Co. 1988. "AIDS Five-Year Comprehensive Service Plan." Los Angeles: County of Los Angeles Department of Health Services.
36. Richwald, Gary A., Donald E. Morisky, Garland R. Kyle, Alan R. Kristal, Michele M. Gerber, and Joan M. Friedland. 1988. "Sexual Activities in Bathhouses in Los

Angeles County: Implications for AIDS Prevention Education."1988. *The Journal of Sex Research* 25:2 169–180.

37. Rivera, Rhonda, R. 1987. In *AIDS and the Law,* edited by Harlon L. Dalton, Scott Burns and the Yale AIDS Law Project. New Haven: Yale University Press.

38. Rogers, Martha F. and Walter W. Williams. 1987. "AIDS in Blacks and Hispanics: Implications for Prevention." *Issues in Science and Technology* (Spring): 89–94.

39. Rosenberg, Charles E. 1962. *The Cholera Years: The United States in 1832, 1849, and 1866.* Chicago: University of Chicago Press.

40. Rothstein, Mark A. 1987. In *AIDS and the Law,* edited by Harlon L. Dalton, Scott Burns and the Yale AIDS Law Project. New Haven: Yale University Press.

41. Rowe, Mona J. and Caitlin C. Ryan. 1988 "Comparing State-Only Expenditures for AIDS." *American Journal of Public Health* 78:4 424–431.

42. Sisk, J.E. 1987. "The Costs of AIDS: A Review of Estimates." *Health Affairs* 6:2 5–21.

43. Scitovsky, A.A. and D.P. Rice. 1987. "Estimates of the Direct and Indirect Costs of Acquired Immunodeficiency Syndrome in the United States, 1985, 1986, 1991." *Public Health Reports* 102:1 5–17.

44. Vaid, Urvashi. 1987 "Prisons." In *AIDS and the Law,* edited by Harlon L. Dalton, Scott Burns and the Yale AIDS Law Project. New Haven: Yale University Press.

45. Yarchoan, Robert, Hiroaki Mitsuya and Samuel Broder. 1988. "AIDS Therapies." *Scientific American,* 259:4 110–119.

Chapter 1

Gender, Sexuality and AIDS: Social Responses and Consequences

Beth E. Schneider

WHEN GENDER AND SEXUALITY are placed at the center of an analysis of the social consequences of HIV infection, complex research questions and policy dilemmas emerge. Many of these issues were obscured by the early conceptualization of AIDS as a disease of white Gay (homosexual) men, and further obliterated by the epidemiological discourse on "risk groups." Each of these initial understandings of AIDS foreclosed the recognition of women as possible AIDS patients, and each took for granted, often without sustained analysis, that the vast majority of people with AIDS are men with particular gendered problems and perspectives.

This essay examines three areas of current and possible research, in which questions about the relationship of sexuality and gender to AIDS, and the social impact on gender and sexual relations of AIDS emerge most clearly. In the first section, the focus is on whether *AIDS has made an impact on sexual talk and behavior* for heterosexual women and men in the past seven years, a concern which invariably addresses the problematic features of AIDS-prevention strategies. Then, some of the unique, male-centered problems generated by HIV infection among IV drug users and Gay men are explored. Finally, the particular social, sexual, and reproductive problems posed for women who are HIV infected are examined. Given the current paucity of of social science research on AIDS (Ergas, 1987), particularly in these areas, this paper focuses on what seems to be known, relying when necessary on suggestive but often unsystematic evidence, and issues and questions for research are offered.

In this analysis of the ways people and institutions deal with AIDS, I am taking as a given certain conceptions about the meaning of gender. Gender refers to both cultural ideals and behavioral practices. Gender differences are socially constructed and socially reproduced. Concepts of gender are cultural interpretations of sex differences that emerge in strongly held beliefs about appropriate, valued behavior in men and women that shape, but do not totally determine, the ways males and females act as gendered persons and the ways they interact with one another. Gender is not static, but flexible, and its meaning becomes clear in the beliefs that people hold and in the context of situated social interaction, where those beliefs are manifested and enacted (Risman, 1987).

Considerable evidence exists that people still hold to the the view that the attributes of women and men are polar opposites; homosexuals are assumed by many to possess the attributes of the other biological sex (Deaux and Kite, 1987). Individuals do not just think in opposites; they do gender in their ordinary, ongoing events and activities in everyday life. Gender is a property of social situations, "a socially organized achievement," (West and Zimmerman, 1987:129) done in interaction with others. Finally, the doing of gender interactionally is linked, though not inevitably, to the social relations of gender in this society which are hierarchically organized, resting on, and resulting in, inequalities of social power and control over labor, resources and services.

AIDS and Sexual Behavior Among Heterosexuals

Alan Brandt (1985:6) in his social history of venereal disease in the United States, argues quite persuasively that "the social and cultural uses of venereal disease as a means of controlling sexuality have greatly complicated attempts to deal effectively with the diseases from a therapeutic standpoint." Brandt demonstrates the ways in which diseases become social symbols for the anxieties and fears of the cultural milieux in which they emerge.

AIDS became public in a political and social terrain in which the issue of changing gender relations and the impact and meaning of a decade's sexual revolution were quite controversial. AIDS, as a medical issue, rapidly became joined, as a structural and social problem, to already heated debate about sexual privacy, reproductive freedom, the viability of relationships which were not heterosexually-married and monogamous, and sex education.

AIDS and the politics surrounding it raises questions about sexual pleasure, sexual talk, sex education, sexual fantasy, sexual practices, sexual identity, sexual community, and sexual regulation. Though social science research in these areas is riddled with methodological flaws that can make findings suspect (Schneider and Gould, 1987), there is overwhelming evidence that in each of these domains, women and men differ markedly in sexual experience and attitude. Nevertheless, "the relationship between gender and sexuality has not been systematically explored" (Schneider and Gould, 1987:124).

Sexual arrangements are socially constructed, historically and culturally contingent. Hence, in thinking about gender and AIDS, it is fair to argue that this epidemic has indeed heightened the salience of sex and sexuality in the culture (Ergas, 1987). We know that AIDS has already produced significant effects on sexual practice among male homosexuals (Rosen, 1986; McKusick, 1986) and altered significantly the quality and type of sexual talk within Gay and Lesbian communities. Certainly media coverage of Gay male sexual practice has recognized its existence and somewhat demythologized it. The ongoing and potentially disastrous effects of AIDS seem to have pressured the media to a reconsideration of what is culturally permissible as indicated by the slow lifting of the ban on condom advertising on television (Aiken, 1987; Patton, 1985). Indeed, the media resistance may always have been greater than the public's disapproval. In 1987, sixty percent of U.S. adults, a majority in all age groups but those over sixty-five, approve of this advertising, and even larger proportions approve of it to prevent the spread of AIDS (Harris, 1987). Most do not believe the ads will offend them, and most believe that the advertising will encourage adolescents to use this form of contraception. This permission-giving has its critical dimension: a majority believe that television has long given the impression that sex is "all fun and no risk" (Harris, 1987).

Have Sexual Scripts Changed?

But, with the exception of Gay men, discussed in the next section, what has actually happened in the sexual realm to heterosexuals since 1981? Has anything changed? For the sociologist of sexuality, the question can be framed simply: have sexual scripts changed in this AIDS crisis? More specifically, has there been any change in who is appropriate as a partner, in what possible acts are done, in when and where sex occurs and, finally, in why people engage in sex and what meanings it has for them (Gagnon, 1977).

The mass media has been relatively consistent in arguing that the "sexual revolution" has come to an end, that the fear of AIDS has or will circumscribe sexual behavior (Smilgis, 1987). This is a claim unsupported by available statistics, one embedded either in a nostalgic yearning for a joyous, uncomplicated pre-AIDS past or in a punitive judgment on its excesses. But considerable doubt should exist for most heterosexuals about their risk and their need to practice safer sex. In the last year, the reading and viewing public has been bombarded with controversial and contradictory reports about the risks of heterosexual sex (Masters, Johnson, Kolodny, 1988; Gould, 1988; Edwards, 1987; Leishman, 1987). This very inconsistency about the degree of risk is, in itself, an impediment to effective preventive education (Fineberg, 1988; Aiken, 1987).

No systematic evidence currently exists to demonstrate behavioral changes in dating practices of heterosexual teenagers or young, unmarried adults. Opinion polls do suggest that AIDS might be having some effect. For example, in a recent Gallup study (1987), one-half of the teens reported that fear of AIDS has "somewhat" affected their social and dating habits. Also, awareness of sex as a transmission route has consistently increased in sexually active heterosexuals (Fineberg, 1988). The ancedotal material in magazines and newspapers also hints at the possibility of change. Tales abound of individuals who practice more foreplay, who are more monogamous, who are celibate rather than engage in casual sex. Suspicion of bisexual men is purportedly on the increase. Some are choosing what they themselves admit might be "inappropriate" partners: married men and "old flames" (Stein, 1987). Some single women, acknowledging their concern about AIDS, report greater discrimination in selecting partners, many choosing to date recently divorced men from long marriages. All this while the singles bar business is booming (Dougherty, 1988).

However, no changes seem evident in the rates of sexual intercourse among the young. While aware of transmission routes, teens have made little change in their behavior as a consequence (Parachini, 1988). Certainly abstinence, even where you might expect to find it, seems missing. For example, a survey done by the evangelical churches for their own purposes revealed that thirty-five percent of the practicing evangelical teenagers have had sexual intercourse by the age of seventeen, compared to fifty-six percent in the rest of the population (*Los Angeles Times,* February 6, 1988). There is some hint that college students may have changed the number of their sexual partners but not their sexual practices. Among the "somewhat affected" adolescents, sixty-five percent believe the pill is the most appropriate contraception for them compared to twenty-seven percent who selected condoms (Gallup, 1987), and while the sexually active adults agree that they should carry condoms, the frequency of their sexual activity has not changed and most fail to use condoms (Fineberg, 1988). Finally, in most large states, the reported cases of syphilis are on the rise suggesting continued unprotected sex.

Social scientists are in no position to assess the meaning of these changes; comparative data from earlier decades on anything approximating a representative sample of the population do not exist or are unavailable (Booth, 1988). And most efforts to chart changes invariably rely on the Kinsey studies whose validity is especially suspect for the younger segments of the population. Even if such knowledge of changes in frequency in practice and partners were available, it is highly unlikely, given the nature of survey research, that any sense of the lived experience and dilemmas of those sexual beings would be revealed (Schneider and Gould, 1987).

AIDS Prevention Issues Differ for Men and Women

AIDS raises all sorts of questions about the ability of people to change their sexual practices and it nicely illustrates that there is no absolute rule of social conditioning. AIDS prevention issues have revealed how very contradictory and difficult questions of gender and sexuality actually are. Sexual negotiations among young heterosexuals will invariably continue to be a particularly complex arena affected by AIDS.

Theoretically, asking people to change their sexual interactions as well as their sexual practice requires a deep understanding of, and a deep empathy for, the socially constructed nature of those interactions and behaviors as well as the meanings of the actors involved. Sex does not exist in a vacuum. The traditional sexual scripts are heterosexual ones and highly gendered, resting on dichotomous notions of male and female sexuality (Gagnon, 1977; Laws and Schwartz, 1977). For the man, the script presupposes that he always wants and is ready for sex, that sex is centered in his orgasm, and that no pleasure is possible without intercourse. He initiates sex, he separates sex from emotions.

Conversely, in the traditional scripts, women deny their sexuality, learn not to be sexual, and don't talk about sex. Women don't initiate sexual encounters and they combine sexuality and intimacy. A woman's sexuality is for something or someone else, never for her own pleasure. There is sufficient evidence to assert that the status of these scripts has changed; nevertheless, elements of them are deeply embedded features of the ways women and men do gender in their sexual relations, and these injunctions are reproduced, often with remarkable emotion, in the ordinary interactions of sexual people.

For example, before AIDS, talking about sex was highly encouraged in sexual advice on talk shows and in how-to books. Talking about sex, including sexual histories and sexual diseases, is even more urgently stressed now. Yet, talking about sex is a primary taboo for most contemporary women (Webster, 1984; Laws and Schwartz, 1977). And, the practice of talk lags far behind these injunctions. Research from sex educators and surveys of sexual attitudes and behaviors find such talk in short supply in the population at any age (Schneider and Gould, 1987). Other studies of sexual interactions among married couples find that the language, hers and his, used to discuss sex often confuses and mystifies communication (Rubin, 1976). Anecdotal evidence, consistent with these other findings, indicates that it is not just AIDS which is going undiscussed, but past partners and past or present sexually transmitted diseases. Medical doctors are still looking for a way to do short, sexual histories which will not embarass them (*New York Times,* 1/9/88). Moreover, our language does not have a selection of good words to describe what we do. We have scientific language ("sexual intercourse"), slang ("fuck"), and euphemisms ("make love"); most talk about sex, especially slang, is accomplished by men, using language created by men (Schneider and Gould, 1987).

AIDS makes this silence much less possible. The universal opinion of sex and health educators calls for direct, clear, explicit discussion of sex and sexual practices in language compatible with the values of specific cultural and sexual communities (National Academy of Sciences, 1986; Aiken, 1987). And at least for Gay men and adult heterosexuals, this effort has been reflected in safer sex guidelines. Most of these materials tend to deromanticize sexual acts; particularly for young women, the message runs counter to an adolescent sexual ideology that emphasizes spontaneity and the link between romance and sex (Luker, 1975; Thompson, 1984).

Safe sex issues are nothing new, especially for women engaged in heterosexual sex. Women have consistently to attend to the matter of pregnancy, and recently to other sexually transmitted diseases which are particularly harmful to women. The majority of condom purchasers are now female (Patton, 1987). There seems little doubt that women are worried about something — preventing pregnancy, STDs (Sexually Transmitted Diseases), AIDS — and that heterosexual women are more concerned about AIDS than heterosexual men.

Again, there is little systematic evidence to indicate what troubles women encounter when they introduce condoms into a sexual scene or talk about changing sexual practice. This introduction of a change in sexual terms necessarily reveals the structured nature of gender in sexual relations; indeed, the distribution of power in erotic activity is another way of studying gender inequality (Schneider and Gould, 1987:125). Much of the prevention material urges women to be even more responsible for sex than they were in the past, locating women as controllers of men's sexuality. Gender is revealed at every turn: Secretary of Education Bennett urges young people, especially women, to be "modest"; if they cannot be modest, then mandatory testing, as a kind of punishment, is proposed (Guardian, 1987). Likewise, Kaplan's book, written for women, (1987) suggests that women simply not be sexual with men until the men are tested. Indeed, two of the four recent books about AIDS expressly for women base their arguments on the belief that men are not to be trusted in sexual matters (Kaplan, 1987; Norwood, 1987).

Whatever the viewpoint toward men, women's sexual partners are an issue in any prevention strategy. What is being asked of women could be dangerous to them since it raises the possibility of domestic, if not cultural, conflict. The age groups most affected by AIDS are precisely those that never had to negotiate male-centered contraception. Young women face the prospect of buying condoms and no one using them. Young women also face the prospect of sexual partners who are sex and drug experimenters; sex with other young men may be part of the rituals and humiliations of youth, and sex with prostitutes may be an initiation into manhood and a consistent sexual outlet for men in the military. Ancedotal accounts from women with AIDS or female partners of HIV-infected men do indicate that some have experienced violence by their partners when they tried to raise the issue of safer sex and the use of condoms (Patton, 1985; Richardson, 1988). In general, women have not been in the best positions to demand compliance from their men. Can women refuse their partners in the AIDS crisis any better than in more normal times?

While this kind of negotiating is inevitable for the vast majority of heterosexuals, it may be particularly complicated in racial/ethnic communities, where unique family and cultural values enter in. For example, Black men seem particularly disdainful of condoms; men who use them are not male enough. Particularly, but certainly not exclusively in Black and Latin communities, many men have sex with men but do not identify themselves as homosexual or even bisexual (Worth and Rodriguez, 1987; Hammonds, 1987). Many female partners of men from Latino communities may not be aware of the homosexual practice of some portion of those men, given cultural prescription against such practices. Moreover, they see the men as superior to them, won't talk about sex—since good women don't—and they defer to men in decision-making related to sex. Being prepared for sex may violate not only Church dictate but their sense of proper womanhood, and cast them as loose and immoral (Worth and Rodriguez, 1987).

An additional consideration in this web of gender and sexuality issues is the ways in which homophobia may structure men's responses to AIDS. Males show consistently higher rates of homophobia than females; white, teen, and college-aged males are the perpetrators of assaults against Lesbians and Gay men (Berrill and Burns, 1984). Homophobia, coupled with the belief in immortality and invincibility among young men, seemingly accounts for the resistance of heterosexual males to efforts at education. These men are particularly likely to joke about sex, including Gay sex, to prove they are "normal" heterosexuals; this defensiveness supports only certain conceptions of manhood. The fear of not being "man enough" is reflected in condom marketing strategies that take into account men's insecurities about their penis size and use slogans such as "Are you man enough for safe sex" or "I like my Miller Lite and my condom tight" to equate the wearing of condoms with being a man (Goldsmith, 1988; Richardson, 1988). While market researchers have recognized this impediment, sex and health educators have yet to note explicitly other possibly powerful fears: that changes in sexual practices for heterosexual men may require the abandonment of expectations of totally spontaneous sex and sexual practices that include penetration.

Homophobia also results in the denial that AIDS has anything to do with them. Even the national media argue that it is precisely the young, heterosexual male who is most indifferent to the disease and its implications for him (Smilgis, 1987). No major AIDS campaign has insisted on the responsibility of heterosexual men in sexual activity.

Research Agenda

Research is necessary to understand what makes change in the sexual realm. As the history of sexually transmitted diseases makes clear, fear alone seems rarely to foster positive change (Brandt, 1985). An examination of the newest research provides little assurance that extensive and sustained change in sexual practices has occurred, except for Gay men and even then only under certain conditions (Fineberg, 1988). As Ergas (1987:36) has suggested, "The belief that information or education suffices to affect behavior is seriously open to question." Differences in the meanings of sexuality for women and men create deep resistance to change. If prevention strategies are to effect the permanent changes virtually everyone argues are needed, they must necessarily grapple not only with issues of cultural sensitivity, but with the complex ways in which gender and sexuality are related. Thus far, it has been only the organized community of Gay men which has developed educational models that take full account of the meanings connected to sexuality in efforts to transform it (Altman, 1987).

A social science research agenda that attempted to grapple with some of these issues would necessarily include, among other things: (1) national, representative panel study of the sexual practices of heterosexual adults, oversampled for the most sexually active (those between 20 and 40) and racial and cultural groups; (2) systematic study of the sexual practices and the meanings of sexuality to adolescents; (3) review and rigorous evaluation of existing sex education programs to assess the extent to which they work — that is, with an eye not only to how information is conveyed and how long it is retained (a common approach), but to how that information is used over the long-term; (4) and qualitative, if not case, analyses of expressions of homophobia among men, extending from violence toward Gay men and Lesbians to its more subtle forms.

Men and HIV Infection

Ninety-two percent of the patients with AIDS in the United States are male. As with some chronic diseases, it is absolutely appropriate to consider the unique, male-centered social problems generated by HIV infection. Much of the research on psychosocial issues in the treatment of AIDS does not discuss these men as gendered persons with possibly unique problems or unique means of coping.

While conceptions of gender have changed and the doing of maleness is more varied than several decades ago, some activities and domains are understood as more or less masculine or feminine, and males and females approximate these understandings in their behavior. The male as a good provider (Bernard, 1981) and the man who heads the household and earns an income for his family remain with us even now. This conception entails not just laboring but also sociological and psychological dimensions — a marked identification of male with work and of success at work with manliness, a limited time for personal interaction and intimacy, and a considerable lack of expressivity (Bernard, 1981; Rubin, 1976). The real man is obviously heterosexual; the real man is a sexual initiator. The real man does not seek much assistance, seeking help is stigmatizing. Indeed, men seek assistance less often than women for mental and physical health problems, including drug use, where men have a proportionally lower rate than women of entrance into treatment.

What is the relationship of these gender expectations to the ways men act, that is "do gender," in an AIDS epidemic? Some of the possible sexual issues of heterosexual men were discussed above. In this section, other concerns which touch on dimensions of manhood, and the doing of gender, are explored for Gay men and the male IV drug user.

Gay Men

Thus far, most of the medical, pyschological and social effects of AIDS in the United States can be most clearly seen in what is written about or by Gay men. With the exception of dealing with the management of sexual identity, many of the personal consequences necessarily affect other persons with AIDS similarly: dealing with illness in the prime of life, deaths of loved ones, managing wide-ranging threats to civil liberties, livelihoods, and shelter. This analysis focuses on only three of the consequences to Gay men: changes in sexual practices, altered interpersonal relationships, and confrontations with death. In each of these areas, the meaning and practice of gender is revealed.

Changes in sexual practices

The Gay male sexual lifestyle of the 1970s affirmed sex outside of relationships and sexual adventure as a positive good. The highly structured commercial, urban, Gay milieu facilitated the possibilities of behavior consistent with these values. This was a male, not a female, world since the commercialization of sex has always been predominantly controlled by and for men (Altman, 1982). Its development occurred in a historical context of social, religious, and legal discrimination, which tend to foster internalized homophobia (Adam, 1978) and is coterminous with the advent of highly political local and national communities of Lesbians and Gay men (Altman, 1986). This combination of factors had consequences for individual identity, community activity, and sexual behavior (Foster, 1988; Epstein, 1987). As Kayal (1986) argues, "At no time can Gay male sexual behavior be understood outside the interaction of sexism, male eros, homophobia, and minority status."

This image and philosophy of sex as an end in itself was coupled with eroticism based on glorification of the beautiful body and its instrumentality. It has been applied to descriptions of Gay men by insiders and outsiders alike; rarely were these descriptions of sexual activity linked to their role in human relationships. Interestingly enough, the homophobia that fueled the early conceptualizations of AIDS ignored the fact that these men were "merely mirroring male socio-sexual expectations" (Kayal, 1986:6), that is, the masculinist basis of Gay male culture and values looked a lot like the ideology of male sexuality.

Hence, considerations of Gay male sexual behavior have been plagued by two particularly glaring problems: the denial of reported research differences among male homosexuals in sexual practice, relationship commitment, way of living (Bell and Weinberg, 1978); and the assumption that male sexual behavior is specialized, independent activity devoid of emotions, feelings, or community attachments. These misperceptions of Gay men, and the presumption that individual sexual acts were all there was to being Gay, found their way into behavioral models implicit in early suggestions for safe sex guidelines. Such models presumed a belief that desires are non-social and hence can be easily altered, indeed without much passion, by acts of will generated through reason and conditioning.

But these assumptions are a poor substitute for sociological thinking about the ways sexuality (for everyone) is linked to social and structural features of the society. The always-sexually-ready male is, as Kayal argues, "An epiphenomenon...a function of the way maleness is defined in our society and historically in the Gay community itself" (Kayal, 1986:14). And cross-cultural research suggests that the majority culture has also contributed to certain components of male homosexual behavior: homophobic attitudes in the majority population are correlated with decreases in long-term coupling among male homosexuals. A society that condemns open and loving relationships between Gay couples seems to encourage closeted, fleeting sexual encounters.

If we consider what has and has not changed for Gay men in the sexual realm, many of the linkages between ways of doing gender in sexual relations and community interests are revealed. The AIDS crisis has seemingly transformed Gay male sexual practice; at the aggregate level, Gay men, if sexual at all, have fewer sexual partners and less often engage in unsafe sexual practices (McKusick, Horstman and Coates, 1986; Rosen, 1986). Though changes are most dramatic for nonsteady partners and unprotected anal sex, not everyone changes. These reductions are most evident when there are high concentrations of AIDS cases and when there is a well-organized Gay community that provides social support and alternative ways of being sexual (Fineberg, 1988). While the virtue of sexual adventure has tarnished, the prospect of pleasurable sex has not. The Gay male press is now full of advertisements for condoms, eroticized massages, and phone sex. Non-genital stimulation is encouraged in "safer sex" guidelines produced by the Gay community.

Altered interpersonal relationships

Ethnographic accounts note that Gay men discuss commitment, intimacy, and monogamy when they talk about relationships — concerns typically attributed to their female counterparts (Altman, 1987). Gay men, even those with diagnosed cases of AIDS, are entering partnerships with other men (Callen, 1988). What has been changed suggests a pragmatic approach to avoiding the spread of AIDS, coupled with a transformation of the terms of being sexual — changes which resonate somewhat with the plea of one, among many, Gay AIDS activists to "learn to love, accept and express the feminine" (Kayal, 1986:26): that is, do gender differently.

In addition, virtually everything written about the experience of Gay men with AIDS reveals a heightened acknowledgment of the need (probably always felt but less often expressed) for support from family and friends (Macks and Turner, 1986; Mandel, 1986). Families of Gay men have demonstrated a spectrum of responses from outright rejection to total support (Interrante, 1987; Macks and Turner, 1986). Social science research has yet to be done that attempts to account for the variability of family support and the creation of kin structures of partners, friends, and children within the Gay male community. The dealing with death as an extended family matter, especially in the face of the lack of legal and psychological support, is worthy of sustained investigation.

Confrontations with Death

Numerous first-person accounts of the impact of AIDS suggest that Gay men, especially those situated in thriving Lesbian/Gay communities, have integrated the immediacy of death into daily life. This, too, has meant an increased appreciation of the meanings and the work involved in nurturing and caregiving. For some Gay men, an AIDS diagnosis is their first experience of getting psychological support and giving care to another (Foster, 1988; Mandel, 1986). In one account (Interrante, 1987), the author illustrates the psychological and emotional growth both men in a Gay partnership experience in facing the impeding death of one of them. Interrante equates this experience as the partner of a man with AIDS with the best of mothering activities: unconditional love, physical caregiving, and an investment in the processes of growth, change, and separation. In this formulation, Interrante suggests that dealing with death is, itself, a gendered event based in differences between men and women in their experiences of their bodies and in the birthing of children. And surely, the most public manifestation of the loss and grieving surrounding AIDS within the Lesbian/Gay community, the "AIDS Quilt," reflects an appreciation of the value of compassion and the powerful symbolic and real work involved in the handicrafts typically made by women.

In all three of these areas, the changes that are occurring for Gay men emphasize ways of doing gender typically attributed to women. With most of the research on Gay men focused on the psycho-social and medical, other social scientists might attempt to do research on the possible meanings to Gay men of these changes and how they have occurred. And finally, ethnographic and socio-historical research is needed on the profound impact of AIDS on the politics, infrastructure, and interpersonal relationships of the Lesbian/Gay community.

Male IV Drug Users

Rarely does the research on male IV drug users consider their lives as men. Unlike the Gay males, analysis of these men rarely begin to touch directly on issues of gender but focuses instead on a matrix of race or class factors.

Characteristics

The majority of male IV (intravenous) drug users are White, and some are middle class. There is, however, a disproportionate number in Black and Latin communities; for example, approximately forty percent of all male IV drug users are Black. National estimates put the number of IV drug users at 900,000 regular users (at least once at week) and 200,000 additional occasional users. Overall, twenty-five percent are HIV-infected; in New York and New Jersey, the estimated rates are closer to seventy percent.

IV drug users are frequently characterized as alienated, antisocial, economically poor, and without social support systems and personal ties (O'Neill, 1987; Z. Foster, 1988). There is no question that IV drug users are less well-organized politically than Gay men, as indeed their communities are less well-organized to deal with AIDS. This characterization is the case for some significant, but seemingly unknown, portion of this population. And yet the cultural stigmatization and denigration of the IV drug user allows the view of a crazed heroin addict infected with dirty needles in the streets of New York to take precedence over the image of a possible, or past drug user and/or a member of a family or parent to a young child (Des Jarlais et al., 1986).

Given the demographics of IV drug use, many of these men probably have failed to validate their own cultural (whether Black, Latino, or Anglo) expectations for men as fathers, husbands, or sexual partners. How could it be otherwise when, for example, the status of Black males between fifteen and twenty-four, never good, has deteriorated badly in the last twenty-five years in terms of rates of unemployment, school attendance, homicide, and drug use. And yet, drug dealing, as well as using, is a way to earn a living for economically marginal families. Dealing is common in poor New York Latino communities (Worth and Rodriguez, 1987), and the drug industry has created lucrative jobs for young Black men in many urban areas across the country. Understanding these men, and their reactions to AIDS, may require accepting the fact that drug dealing is one means to avoid failure as a man in low-income communities.

There is a high turnover among IV drug users (Waldorf and Biernachi, 1981; Robins, 1980). Each year, approximately ten to twenty percent leave the stable-user population, and these are replaced usually by new users. Lower-class heroin addicts begin to outgrow addiction with adulthood, with most inactive by their mid-thirties. The paths out of addiction vary: some addicts turn to other drugs, some end the hustling, some simply give it up. Here, similar to the failure of techniques to change sexual behavior, prior research evidence indicates that fear of consequences, including possibly contracting AIDS, does not prevent young men from experimenting. In New York City, AIDS has not become a primary reason to avoid drug injections (Des Jarlais et al., 1988).

Adolescents in many racial and cultural communities are at risk for HIV infection, at least in part, because the desire for peer acceptance leads to drugs and sex. It is impossible to avoid the conclusion that the socio-economic conditions that constrain the lives of these men are at issue in any serious effort to think about prevention of AIDS in urban areas not already facing epidemic proportions of infected IV drug users.

The Prospect of an AIDS Death

Death, through overdose, was always a possibility in drug use subcultures (Des Jarlais et al., 1988). Death from AIDS is different from facing the prospect of the overdose: Death from AIDS is protracted and painful; it opens the possibility of complex and potentially disrupted social interaction with drug users' friends and family, both of whom, according to Des Jarlais and his associates, fear casual contact. While some commentators assume that they will "...refuse to consider using safe practices" (Z. Foster, 1988), IV drug users in some urban areas seem to be altering their risk of contracting AIDS through changes in needle-using practices (O'Neill, 1987). The changes that have thus far been reported were prior to any prevention campaigns begun in New York and, hence, seem to represent the workings of the informal networks within the subculture (Des Jarlais et al., 1988). As yet, there seems to be no published ethnographic accounts of the ways in which the IV drug-use subculture, with its structured interpersonal networks of "running partners," is making these adjustments to the facts of AIDS.

Interestingly, and contrary to most notions about the male IV drug user, research on these men and AIDS reveals that some male IV drug users face these unpleasant alternatives and choose to deepen relationships, reconcile with families, and search for new meanings in their lives. A diagnosis seems to elicit the desire to regain health and enter treatment. Researchers note that the stress of the diagnosis is positive, resulting in a great deal of courage among the IV drug users and their families in dealing with AIDS (Des Jarlais et al., 1988).

However, not all the research on IV drug users shows this pattern. Another study reported by France (1988) on ex-addicts reveals a more complex reaction. The behavior of ex-addicts seems to vary depending on whether or not they know their antibody status. Those who know they are seropositive tend to return to drug use, seemingly preferring the possibility of death by overdose to death by AIDS. But those who are unaware of their status or test negative continue in drug treatment. Once again, the complexities of these issues are revealed and further research is needed to sort out these dynamics. Findings such as these play havoc with any social policy that advocates mandatory testing for this group.

For both treatment and prevention, the notion of being a man, and the resources by which to accomplish manliness, are at issue for the male IV drug user. Future social science research on AIDS and male IV drug users requires that distinctions among these men be drawn in terms of their relationship to drugs (the ex-addict, recreational user, regular, long-term user) so that the basis on which they respond to either education or AIDS treatment can be fully understood. Moreover, most of the current published research has been conducted in New York City; future work must be done in other urban settings where drug use cultural patterns differ and rates of infection are currently low.

HIV-Infected Women

Eight percent of diagnosed AIDS cases in this country are among women. Without attention to the complex ways in which gender, class, and race intersect (Collins, 1986), it is next to impossible to understand the particular situation of the majority of HIV-infected women. AIDS among females necessarily points to specific issues concerning a host of reproductive, sexual, and family issues that simply do not emerge clearly when the focus is on men. Women with AIDS do not fit into the male AIDS profiles since the latter inadequately address some of the central physiological or sociopolitical differences between women and men, and fail to situate these women in their own unique historical and material conditions which shaped their lives.

Drug use accounts for fifty percent of the female AIDS cases. But the proportion of women getting AIDS from male sexual partners has more than doubled in five years (from twelve percent in 1982 to twenty-six percent in 1986). Seventy percent of the women with AIDS are Black and Latino and, of the total, over half reside in the New York/New Jersey metropolitan area and Florida. In New York City, AIDS is now the major cause of death in women twenty-five to twenty-nine. Immediately two general questions emerge: how do women cope with the still-prevalent view that AIDS is a male disease?; and how do women of color cope with the still-prevalent view that AIDS is a white person's disease?

Women with AIDS: Neither Male, nor Gay, nor White

The female AIDS patients do not, in any obvious sense, constitute a self-conscious, politically active community. The small proportion of women thus far with AIDS, and their diversity, creates a "disease of isolation" (Cimons, 1988). Moreover, most of the women currently at highest risk or with AIDS, given their demographic and social profile, are least likely to have access to adequate medical care or health insurance. The public, to the extent that it has awareness of these women, no doubt can easily scapegoat intravenous drug users and poor women of color. Unfortunately, minority women of childbearing age are frequently considered, for reasons that are rarely spelled out in the AIDS literature, "a hard-to-reach population" (Edwards, 1987). It may well be that this notion is based on a stereotype of Black women as uneducated and lacking in the facts for sound judgment, rather than reflective of particular ways in which they face the nature of their oppression (Collins, 1987). More generally, women typically may encounter blaming-the-victim responses to their sexuality, pregnancies, abortions, sexually transmitted diseases, and prostitution (Buckingham and Rehm, 1987).

This blaming was clear in the early cultural and medical panic about prostitutes spreading AIDS (see, for example, Redfield et al., 1986), a claim which was only recently proven to be unwarranted in most cases by the recently published *Prostitute Study* published by Centers for Disease Control. It reveals that, with the exception of New York, New Jersey, and Florida, where the general incidence of AIDS is very high and the incidence among IV drug users is even higher, the incidence of HIV infection among prostitutes tends to be quite low. In the only study using a control group, prostitutes showed no higher rate of infection than a matched group of sexually active women, when the data was adjusted for other risk factors (U.S. Centers for Disease Control, 1987). Prostitutes and other women are already at risk as a result of the men with whom they are involved ("johns," bisexual and homosexual men, drug users), yet they, and not their clients, are likely to be stigmatized and blamed for their real and imagined sexual activities (Shaw and Paleo, 1986; Richardson, 1988).

In addition, the life conditions and social-psychological stresses for women (especially those with children) differ markedly from those of most men, especially White homosexual men about whom most research concerning AIDS has been undertaken and for whom most services concerning AIDS are organized. And all social-psychological dimensions which have an impact on stress (coping strategies, role strain, life events, and social support) are theoretically constructed differently for each racial/ethnic group (Kaplan, 1983). Even medically, the women with AIDS are different. Early in the epidemic, HIV-infected women were misdiagnosed. On the aggregate, women are dying faster than men. White Gay men with Karposki's Sarcoma only, had the best survival rates; Black IV drug-using women had the worst (*New England Journal of Medicine,* November 19, 1987:1297-1302). It is not yet clear whether Gay men live longer after a diagnosis with AIDS because the pattern of disease is different or because they seek care earlier. But what is clearer is that the results of expanding drug trials may not be valid for women, as well as all drug users, if AIDS is manifested differently among them (Kolata, 1988).

Pregnancy and Motherhood

Feminist scholars have long noted that pregnancy and childhood are medicalized events which minimize the social, emotional, and psychological aspects of motherhood (Rothman, 1987). AIDS threatens to further medicalize each of these processes by creating further conditions under which women are passive recipients of medical services. In what has been written thus far on women with AIDS, the medical profession's tendency to view women in terms of their unique reproductive capacities has held sway. That is, there is intervention where women are unique but minimization of women's problems where men have similar problems (Zimmerman, 1987). Hence, in research on women with AIDS, a pattern exists similar to that already applied to female drug users, which focuses on health effects as they pertain primarily to pregnancy and neonates, with little to no attention to the broader contours of these women's lives.

It is crucially important in understanding women with AIDS to recognize this issue of motherhood. Eighty percent of the children with AIDS acquired it through their mothers who have AIDS or are HIV-infected. And the possibility of pediatric AIDS does raise innumerable issues for women. There are so many unknowns when it comes to pediatric AIDS. The method by which AIDS is transmitted from mother to infant remains unclear (National Academy of Sciences, 1986), and transmission of the virus does not occur in all pregnancies of seropositive women. At the present moment, most women are unaware of their antibody status. Medical research suggests that for women infected with HIV, pregnancy increases their own chances of developing AIDS. And the child of an AIDS infected mother has a considerable risk of being infected (Pinching and Jeffries, 1985; National Academy of Sciences, 1986). However, not all babies infected will develop AIDS. These unknown factors must necessarily affect women who plan to be or are already pregnant, though, at present, it is not clear how.

Women, especially those at some risk, have been urged to postpone pregnancy until researchers learn more about the significance of a positive antibody test, the relationship between pregnancy and symptom development, and the risk of infection to the newborn infant. Wise as this may seem, the decision to forego pregnancy or terminate a pregnancy is typically not made lightly for most women. All women, whatever their cultural heritage, confront issues in the AIDS epidemic about control over their reproductive futures and sexual desires, the meaning of children for them, values concerning abortion, and the inevitable confrontation with the biological time clock. The distributions of unplanned pregnancies and sexually transmitted diseases parallel one another, revealing a highly structured sexual stratification in the society (Cates, 1984; Darrow, 1977). Situational opportunities often determine women's decisions about childbearing. These issues have varying significance and impact among women of different class and racial backgrounds.

More specifically, Black teenagers are more sexually active than Whites, less likely to use contraception and abortion, and the Black proportion of out-of-wedlock births is higher (National Center for Health Statistics, 1982; Zelnick and Kanter, 1980). The result of these trends is that one out of two Black children are born to mothers who are not married. These facts, in part, reflect historically different views of the value of children and Black community support of single motherhood (O'Connell, 1980; Thompson, 1980), and in part, they reflect the interlocking structures of race and class oppression.

For women with ARC (AIDS Related Complex) or AIDS, their activities as primary parent are utterly transformed. Family patterns are disrupted. Research sensitive to the ways in which the unique kinship patterns common to very poor Black women operate might investigate their resiliency in the face of these extraordinary conditions.

In addition, it is through motherhood that Latinas affirm their status as women, and research on female drug addicts reveals that their children and motherhood are their singular claim to worthiness (Rosenbaum, 1981). Hence, any understanding of motherhood in these women's lives must touch on the choices available to them within opportunity structures, their material conditions, and their perceptions of the possibilities for themselves and their children.

The female drug user

In addition, more research is necessary on female drug users. Until this last decade, there was little research done on these women. Earlier work typically employed information and stereotypes about male users to understand the women. Efforts to understand the relatively smaller number of female users were typically hampered by what Harris describes as "typescripts," deeply rooted "assumptions about *who does what, including deviance,* in a society" (Harris, 1977:3; italics in original). Typescripts affect the labeling and processing of persons as deviant. The typescript for the drug user, the heroin addict, is ambiguous for females. There have always been fewer female users than male, and for the last several decades young drug users have tended to be urban, male members of racial/ethnic groups (Robins, 1980). In addition, the underworld-related distribution network and the typical need among drug-users to commit property crimes to support their habits may have been factors conducive to female-inappropriateness in taking up drugs or to researchers' assumptions about the existence of these women.

The work of Rosenbaum (1981) on female heroin users provides some sense of the contours of these women's lives. Women commonly begin using heroin at later ages than men and become users through introduction to drugs by a man (Worth and Rodriguez, 1987; Rosenbaum, 1981). The women become part of the world of their partner. The heroin life becomes the focal point of their existence, threatening both their occupational options and their love relationships with men. Women's habits are larger than men's in terms of cost and quantity. They are the dependent consumers rather than providers; a sizable number rely on prostitution to earn money to support their habits.

Rosenbaum's study reveals that partners in a couple are usually of similar status, both current or both former addicts. Sexual relations are often absent due to lack of interest and inability to perform. Many women claim that the fixing routines and other aspects of taking heroin together, especially when heroin is administered by their partner, replace sexual intercourse. In the study, drugs killed the relationships; trust eroded as traditional gender expectations were disrupted. Many women were more able to work consistently than men through prostitution, and the differential earnings became a source of conflict: the man resented his dependence, the woman felt exploited.

One of the major differences between male and female addicts lies in their responsibilities, which for the male most often involves heroin-related work, and for the women revolves around the care of their children. A higher percentage of women than men in treatment programs have dependent children. To raise their children, women must rely on many resources including their extended kin. Women experience a conflict between their efforts to attain heroin and their mothering. Women addicts are often violating their own strong moral codes in practicing prostitution. They believe they should be taking care of their children. The female addict's inability to fulfill her mothering responsibilities destroys the non-addict identity that might make escape from "the life" possible.

Women living with AIDS

Given what is known about both the female drug users and the other women at greatest risk of HIV-infection, what does the introduction of AIDS do to their lives? How is a woman with AIDS able to care for her children? And what does she feel about herself and her options? At this point, there is little that social scientists can offer to address these questions. It is primarily from the work of medical practitioners that an outline of the parameters of the situation of these women emerges; careful qualitiative research with these women is needed to provide a detailed understanding of the ways in which they manage, and the meanings women attribute to their illness and to the actions they take as a consequence.

Care of children requires comprehensive, coordinated effort, including the acute care setting, the home and the community. Caretakers need help in coping with the impact of chronic illness on themselves, and possibly their children, as well with family and community response to the label of AIDS. The family requires not only traditional health care services, but assistance with social and educational institutions (Buckingham and Rehm, 1987). Women with a diagnosis of AIDS qualify for federal and state disability payments and for Medicare, but women who are only HIV-infected do not, even though they may be unable to care for their families or continue to work.

With the current trend to shorter hospital stays for AIDS patients, home care becomes a larger concern. And yet, in many instances, the home environment and the family specifically may not be able to provide what the child needs. These are primarily low-income, single-parent families (Shaw and Paleo, 1986). At any one time, mothers who are HIV-infected may or may not be ill themselves; there may be one or more sick children and other uninfected children at home. Questions emerge about the quality of care, about whether protective service agencies have entered, or could enter, the home to make assessment of health neglect. The family members may be quite distrustful of human services and health institutions and their interventions. Moreover, home care will likely be affected by public knowledge about AIDS transmission. While studies of the families of AIDS patients have revealed no instances of transmission to adults who were not sexual partners or to children who were not already at risk at birth (Friedland et.al., 1985), sizable proportions of U.S. adults believe that AIDS can be transmitted casually.

In addition, while it is clear that women are often buffered by social networks that encompass family, friends, and neighbors, and that these networks can be especially useful in troubled circumstances, they may nevertheless exact a toll and be sources of additional stress for these women. Women are often expected to nurture and help people who help them. And while men generally turn to women in times of difficulty, many of these women cannot expect to rely on men; many women suffer a gap in support, giving support to everyone and not getting it in return. This suggests there is a need for a comparative study of racial and cultural variability in support systems to adult women who are diagnosed with AIDS.

Some mothers with AIDS will surely die before their infants and face, while quite ill, significant decisions about what to do about their children. Foster care placement is necessary for the children of these mothers if kin support is unavailable. However, foster care systems in the major metropolitan areas are already overtaxed, and the number of children awaiting such placement is greater than the available homes. It is already the case that Black children primarily are going to be even more disadvantaged in this regard, because families are becoming unwilling to take a healthy child fearing that he or she may be AIDS-infected (Grossman, 1988).

There is a critical need for social and medical services and educational information about AIDS that is accessible and sensitive to women. In addition, women need more of what they already needed before AIDS: drug treatment programs for women with and without children; sustained prenatal care; increased foster care services and child care facilities; confidential counseling at family planning and prenatal clinics; continued access to abortion and state-funded abortions; sex education; national health care in some form; and basic survival provisions in food, clothing, and shelter. In other words, the AIDS crisis reveals, through the lives of women with AIDS, the already serious shortcomings in the health, human services, and educational apparatus in this country. That women with AIDS do not have sufficient access to or control over these resources represents the intersection of gender, race, and class inequalities.

Ethical issues and research questions

AIDS has stimulated wide-ranging discussions about the relationship between civil liberties and public health. Women are in a particularly critical situation in this regard as the implications of some policy proposals force them to confront ethical and rights issues unique to women. There have been recommendations to test all pregnant women and all persons who are seeking to marry. It is quite possible that women or selected groups of them will be the first civilian, non-incarcerated population in the United States to confront mass screening for HIV. Ethically, these plans focus renewed attention to women's rights concerning sex and reproduction: that is, women's rights to control sexual practice, women's rights to privacy, women's rights to sexual and other freedoms, women's rights to be pregnant (Murphy, 1988). AIDS also raises ethical dilemmas for women analogous to those of pregnant women facing decisions about possible births of children with mental and physical disabilities.

The ethical issues have social-scientific parallel questions. What is the decision-making calculus women use or will use to weigh these often competing rights? How have women responded and how will they respond to the threat to confidentiality, if all women at prenatal and birth control clinics are routinely tested? How have women from different backgrounds responded to public messages to curtail sexual activity or forego childbearing, and how will they respond? How do women vary in their response to a possible threat of mandatory abortions for infected pregnant women? What political struggles might ensue among organized groups already concerned with issues such as sex education, abortion, and family planning?

Conclusion

The questions have hardly been asked, let alone the research done, about the impact of AIDS on the social relations of sexuality, on the ways in which individuals do gender, and on the social organization and dynamics of domestic arrangements. In fact, given the early conceptualization of AIDS, it is difficult to think about AIDS and gender.

Nevertheless, this account points to some of the microstructural aspects of gendered behavior at work in an AIDS epidemic. Whatever the group under consideration (Gay or heterosexual men, male or female IV drug users, Black or White women), their behaviors and identities are, as Risman (1987:10) argues, "...circumscribed by the social organization of experiences available" to them. So too, are their responses to AIDS.

AIDS raises questions about the social processes through which women and men, as well as cultural and sexual communities, are engendered. If social science research on the social consequences of AIDS is intended to improve upon medical and simple behavioral models of human activity, particular attention must be paid to the totality of factors shaping people's experiences. The social consequences of AIDS in terms of its impact on gender and sexual relations necessarily demand that research give serious attention to material conditions, opportunity structures, situated social interaction, and locations in social networks, all of which create and sustain the cultural definitions and behavioral repertoires of gendered and sexual persons.

References

1. Adam, Barry. *The Survival of Domination: Inferiorization and Everyday Life.* North Holland: Elsevier. 1978.
2. Aiken, Jane Harris. "Education as Prevention." pp. 90–105 in Dalton, Burris, Scott and Yale AIDS Law Project (eds.), *AIDS and the Law.* New Haven: Yale University Press. 1987.
3. Altman, Dennis. *AIDS in the Mind of America.* New York: Anchor. 1987.
4. ——————.*The Homosexualization of America.* Boston: Beacon. 1982.
5. Bell, A.P. and M. Weinberg. *Homosexualities: A Study of Diversity Among Men and Women.* New York: Simon and Schuster. 1978.
6. Berrill, Kevin and J. Burns. "NGTF Violence Survey Indicates Anti-Gay/Lesbian Violence Widespread." *Task Force Report* New York: National Gay Task Force. vol. 11, no. 2 (March–May 1984):1.
7. Bernard, Jesse. "The Good Provider: Its Rise and Fall." *American Psychologist* 36, 1 (January 1981):1–12.
8. Booth, William. "The Long, Lost Survey on Sex." Science 239:1084–1085.
9. Brandt, Alan. *No Magic Bullet: A Social History of Venereal Disease in the United States Since 1880.* Oxford University Press. 1985.
10. Buckingham, Stephan L. and Susan Rehm. "AIDS and Women at Risk." *Health and Social Work Journal* 12, 1 (Winter 1987):5–11.
11. Callen, Michael. "I Will Survive." *Village Voice* (May 3, 1988):31–35.
12. Cates, William. Jr. "Sexually Transmitted Diseases and Family Planning." *Journal of Reproductive Medicine* 29, 5 (May 1984):317–322.
13. Cimons, Marlene. "For Women, AIDS Brings Special Woes." *Los Angeles Times* (January 8, 1988):1, 12.
14. Collins, Patricia Hill. "Learning from the Outsider Within: The Social Significance of Black Feminist Thought." *Social Problems* 33,6 (December 1986):S14–S32.
15. Darrow, W. W. "Sexual Stratification, Sexual Behavior, and the Sexually Transmitted Diseases." *Sexually Transmitted Diseases* 4 (1977):228–236.
16. Des Jarlais, D., Casriel, C. and S.R.Friedman. "The New Death among IV Drug Users." in I. Corless and M. Pittman-Lindeman (eds.), *AIDS: Principles, Practices, and Politics.* Hemisphere. 1988.
17. Des Jarlais, D. Friedman, S.R. and D. Strug. "AIDS and Needle Sharing within the IV-Drug Use Subculture." in D.A. Feldman and T.A Johnson (eds), *Social Dimensions of AIDS.* Praeger. 1986.
18. Dougherty, Margot. "AIDS and the Single Woman." *People Magazine* (1987):102–105.
19. Edwards, Diane. "Heterosexuals and AIDS: Mixed Messages." *Science News* 132 (July 25, 1987):60–61.

20. Epstein, Stephen. "Gay Politics, Ethnic Identity: The Limits of Social Constructionism." *Socialist Review* 17 (May-August 1987):9–54.
21. Ergas, Yasmine. "The Social Consequences of the AIDS Epidemic." *Social Science Research Council* 41, 3–4 (December 1987).
22. Fineberg, Harvey. "Education to Prevent AIDS: Prospects and Obstacles." *Science* 239 (February 5, 1988):592–596.
23. Foster, Jim. "Impact of the AIDS Epidemic on the Gay Political Agenda." in I. Corless and M. Pittman-Lindeman (eds.), *AIDS: Principles, Practices and Politics*. Washington, D.C.: Hemisphere Publishing. 1988.
24. Foster, Zelda. "The Treatment of People with AIDS: Psychosocial Considerations." in I. Corless and M. Pittman-Lindeman (eds.), *AIDS: Principles, Practices and Politics*. Washington, D.C.: Hemisphere Publishing. 1988.
25. France, D. "Relapses of Recovering Addicts." *Newsday* (May 3, 1988).
26. Friedland, G.H. et al., "Lack of Transmission of HTLV-III/LAV Infection to Household Contacts of Patients with AIDS or AIDS-related Complex With Oral Candidiasis." *New England Journal of Medicine* 314 (February 1985).
27. Gagnon, John. *Human Sexualities*. Glenview, IL: Scott, Foresman. 1977.
28. Gallup, George. "Newsweek Poll on AIDS and Birth Control." Study Number G087049 (February 7, 1987).
29. Goldsmith, Marsha. "Sex in the Age of AIDS Calls for Common Sense and 'Condom Sense'." *Journal of the American Medical Association* 257, 17 (May 1, 1987):2261–2266.
30. Gould, Robert E. "Reassuring News about AIDS: A Doctor Tells Why You May Not Be at Risk." *Cosmopolitan* (January 1988).
31. Grossman, Moses. "Children With AIDS." in I. Corless and M. Pittman-Lindeman (eds.), *AIDS: Principles, Practices and Politics*. Washington, D.C.: Hemisphere Publishing. 1988.
32. *Guardian*. "Falwell Mounts Hysterical Gay-Bashing Campaign." (May 20, 1987):5.
33. Hammonds, E. "Race, Sex, AIDS: The Construction of 'Other'." *Radical America* 20, 6 (1987).
34. Harris, Louis and Associates. "Attitudes About Television, Sex and Contraception." Study No. 874005 (February 1987).
35. Interrante, Joseph. "To Have Without Holding: Memories of Life With a Person With AIDS." *Radical America* 20, 6 (1987).
36. Kaplan, Howard (ed.). *Psychosocial Stress: Trends in Theory and Research*. New York: Academic Press. 1983.
37. Kaplan, Helen Singer. *The Real Truth about Women and AIDS: How to Eliminate Risks Without Giving Up Love and Sex*. New York: Simon and Schuster. 1987.
38. Kayal, Philip M. "Healing Maladaptive Sexual Behavior." Paper presented at the 1986 meetings of the Society for the Study of Social Problems. New York.
39. Kolata, Gina. "AIDS Research on New Drugs Bypasses Addicts and Women." *New York Times* (January 5, 1988):C1.
40. Laws, Judith and Pepper Schwartz. *Sexual Scripts: The Social Construction of Female Sexuality*. Hinsdale, IL: Dryden Press. 1977.

41. Leishman, Katie. "Heterosexuals and AIDS." *Atlantic Monthly* (February 1987).
42. Luker, Kristin. *Taking Chances: Abortion and the Decision Not to Contracept.* Berkeley, CA: University of California Press. 1975.
43. Macks, Judith and Dan Turner. "Mental Health Issues of Persons with AIDS." in L. McKusick (ed.), *What To Do About AIDS: Physicians and Mental Health Professionals Discuss the Issues.* Berkeley, CA: University of California Press. 1986.
44. Mandel, Jeffrey S. "Psychosocial Challenges of AIDS and ARC: Clinical and Research Observations." in L. McKusick (ed.), *What To Do About AIDS: Physicians and Mental Health Professionals Discuss the Issues.* Berkeley, CA:University of California Press. 1986.
45. Masters, W. H., Johnson, V. E. and R.C. Kolodny. *Crisis: Heterosexual Behavior in the Age of AIDS.* New York: Grove Press. 1988.
46. McKusick, L. Horstman, W. and TJ Coates. "AIDS and Sexual Behavior Reported by Gay Men in San Francisco." *American Journal of Public Health* (1986) 75:493-496.
47. Murphy, Angela. "Women with AIDS: Sexual Ethics in an Epidemic." in I. Corless and M. Pittman-Lindeman (eds), *AIDS: Principles, Practices, and Politics.* Hemisphere. 1988.
48. National Academy of Sciences. *Mobilizing Against AIDS.* Cambridge, MA: Harvard University Press. 1986.
49. National Broadcasting Company/*Wall Street Journal.* "January National Poll, Poll Number 122." (January 216, 1987).
50. National Center for Health Statistics. "Monthly Vital Statistics Report." *Advance Report of Final Natality, 1980.* 31, 8 (1982).
51. *New York Times.* "AIDS Testing Without Consent Reported." (January 9, 1988):7.
52. Norwood, Chris. *Advice for Life: A Woman's Guide to AIDS Risks and Prevention.* New York: Pantheon. 1987.
53. O'Connell, M. "Comparative Estimates of Teenage Illegitimacy in the United States, 1940–44 to 1970–74." *Demography* 17 (February 1980):13–24.
54. O'Neill, Catherine. "Intravenous Drug Users." in Dalton, Burris, Scott and Yale AIDS Law Project (eds.), *AIDS and the Law.* New Haven, CT.: Yale University Press. 1987.
55. Parachini, Allan. "AIDS Experts Fear Education Programs are Insufficient." *Los Angeles Times* Part V, pp.1, 13 (March 25, 1988).
56. Patton, Cindy. "Resistance and the Erotic." *Radical America* 20, 6 (1987).
57. Pinching, A. and D. Jeffries. "AIDS and HTLV-III/LAV Infection: Consequences for Obstetrics and Perinatal Medicine." *British Journal of Obstetrics and Gynecology* 92 (1985):1211–1217.
58. Redfield, R.R., et al., "Letter to the Editor." *Journal of the American Medical Association.* 255 (1986):1705–6.
59. Richardson, Diane. *Women and AIDS.* New York: Methuen. 1988.
60. Risman, Barbara J. "Intimate Relationships From a Microstructural Perspective." *Gender and Society* 1, 1 (March 1987):6–32.

61. Robins, Lee. "The Natural History of Drug Abuse." in *Theories of Drug Abuse*. National Institute of Drug Abuse. Washington: U.S. Government Printing. 1980.
62. Rothman, Barbara Katz. "Reproduction." pp.154–189 in Beth Hess and Myra Marx Ferree (eds.), *Analyzing Gender*. Newbury Park, CA:Sage. 1987.
63. Rosen, Don. "LA Gay Men Reduce Unsage Sex Practices, Survey Finds." *Los Angeles Times* (March 21, 1986):1.
64. Rosenbaum, Marsha. *Women on Heroin*. New Brunswick, NJ: Rutgers University Press. 1981.
65. Rubin, Lillian. *Worlds of Pain: Life in the Working-Class Family*. New York: Stein and Day. 1976.
66. Schneider, Beth and Meredith Gould. "Female Sexuality: Looking Back Into the Future." in B. Hess and M.M. Ferree (eds.), *Analyzing Gender*. Sage. 1987.
67. Shaw, N. and Lyn Paleo. "Women and AIDS." in Leon McKusick (ed.), *What To Do About AIDS: Physicians and Mental Health Professionals Discuss the Issues*. Berkeley: University of California Press. 1986.
68. Smilgis, M. "The Big Chill: Fear of AIDS." *Time* (February 16, 1987).
69. Stein, Jeannine. "AIDS Launches the Sexual Counterrevolution." *Los Angeles Times* (April 13, 1987).
70. Thompson, K. "A Comparison of Black and White Adolescents' Beliefs About Having Children." *Journal of Marriage and the Family* 42 (February 1980):133–140.
71. Thompson, Sharon. "Search for Tomorrow: On Feminism and the Reconstruction of Teen Romance." in C. Vance (ed.), *Pleasure and Danger*. Boston: Routledge and Kegan Paul. 1984.
72. United States Centers for Disease Control. "Morbidity and Mortality Weekly Report." (March 13, 1987).
73. Waldorf, D. and P. Biernachi. "The Natural Recovery from Opiate Addiction." *Journal of Drug Issues* 11 (1981):61–74.
74. Webster, Paula. "The Forbidden: Eroticism and Taboo." in C. Vance (ed.), *Pleasure and Danger*. Boston: Routledge and Kegan Paul. 1984.
75. West, Candace and Don Zimmerman. "Doing Gender." *Gender & Society* 1, 2 (June 1987).
76. Worth, Dooley and Ruth Rodriguez. "Latina Women and AIDS." *Radical America* 20, 6 (November 1987).
77. Zelnick, M. and J. Kantner. "Sexual Activity, Contraceptive Use and Pregnancy Among Metropolitan-area Teenagers: 1971–1979." *Family Planning Perspectives* 12 (September–October 1980):230–237.
78. Zimmerman, Mary K. "The Women's Health Movement: A Critique of Medical Enterprise and the Position of Women." pp.442–472 in Beth Hess and Myra Marx Ferree (eds.), *Analyzing Gender*. Newbury Park, CA: Sage. 1987.

Chapter 2

AIDS and the Pornography Industry: Opportunities for Prevention, and Obstacles

Paul Abramson

BETWEEN 1981 AND 1987, nearly 50,000 Americans were diagnosed with Acquired Immunodeficiency Syndrome (AIDS). Of these 50,000 individuals, over half (fifty-six percent) died. Furthermore, the mortality rate of those individuals diagnosed before 1985 is eighty percent (Curran et al, 1988).

Equally dismal are the prospects for a rapid cure or vaccine. The human immunodeficiency virus (HIV), which is responsible for AIDS, exhibits considerable antigenic variation. Moreover, it has been difficult to identify the antibodies that neutralize HIV. Finally, since HIV initiates infection in T cell antigen receptors, which paradoxically are necessary for an effective immune response, immunization runs the risk of harming T cells (Osborn, 1986b).

Consequently, educational intervention is now the primary strategy for diminishing the proliferation of HIV (Fineberg, 1988; Osborn, 1986a, 1986b). This strategy subsumes two initiatives. First, epidemiologic investigations must isolate the transmission dynamics of HIV. Secondly, educational or behavioral interventions must then be designed to effectively prevent transmission.

Presently, it appears that there are three primary modes of HIV transmission: sexual contact (the most likely avenue being rectal trauma during anal intercourse (Kingsley et al., 1987)); parenteral exposure to blood and blood products (principally through sharing contaminated needles or transfusions (Friedland & Klein, 1987)); and vertically (from mother to child during the perinatal period [Curran, et al., 1988]).

Where sexual transmission of HIV is concerned, prevention strategies have focused primarily upon the Gay male population (Grant, Wiley & Winklestein, 1987; McKusic, Hortsman & Coates, 1985; Richwald, et al, 1988). This circumstance is not surprising, since most cases of sexual transmission of HIV have occurred between Gay men (Curran, et al, 1988). Moreover, Gay men are at much higher risk for HIV because they are more likely to engage in anal intercourse, experience rectal trauma, or have multiple sexual partners.

Although Gay men have a greater likelihood of engaging in anal intercourse, the practice of anal intercourse is not limited to Gay men. While experienced much less frequently, anal intercourse is also part of the sexual repertoire of many bisexual and heterosexual couples. Having multiple sexual partners is also by no means predetermined by sexual orientation. Bisexual and heterosexual men and women also initiate non-monogamous relationships. Consequently, researchers have suggested also targeting other high-risk groups, besides Gay men, exhibiting "risky" behaviors (multiple sexual partners, anal intercourse, etc.). Prostitutes (Piot, et al, 1988; *San Francisco Epidemiologic Bulletin,* 1987), Brazil's Carnival participants (Parker, 1987), sexually active college students (Baldwin & Baldwin, 1988), and other groups, have been the subjects of AIDS research and the targets of prevention strategies.

Conspicuously missing from this area of investigation, however, are actors and actresses in the pornography industry. This void is surprising, and perhaps even alarming, since actors and actresses in the pornography industry engage in the entire repertoire of high-risk sexual behaviors (anal intercourse, multiple partners, etc.) as a routine requirement of their profession. Therefore, the purpose of the present chapter is to examine the risks, and strategies for prevention, of HIV infection within the pornography industry.

As an introduction to this subject, the structure of the pornography industry within Los Angeles, California will be described. Los Angeles has been selected for investigation because it is the site of production for nearly eighty percent of American pornography (Attorney General's Commission on Pornography, 1986). This circumstance, incidentally, is a function of favorable political (i.e., liberal) and climatic (i.e., weather) conditions, plus accessibility to technical personnel (camera operators, etc.).

Once the structure of the pornography industry has been articulated, several research perspectives will be introduced, and strategies for initiating AIDS prevention will be discussed. Finally, the opportunities and obstacles for successful intervention will be explored.

Before proceeding however, a number of disclaimers are warranted. First, this chapter ignores the controversy surrounding the impact of pornography (Abramson & Hayashi, 1984; Attorney General's Commission on Pornography, 1986; Malamuth & Donnerstein, 1984; *Technical Report of the Commission on Obscenity and Pornography,* 1971). Furthermore, this chapter does not review legal arguments either supporting or condemning obscenity and sexuality-related materials (Penrod & Linz, 1984; Richards, 1974, 1979, 1983). Instead, the present chapter is intentionally pragmatic and impartial. Hence, the following perspective has been adopted: 1) the pornography industry exists, and 2) pornography actors and actresses warrant strategies to diminish the risk of HIV transmission. Incidentally, this utilitarian approach to pornography is not unique. The pornography industry and the impact of pornographic films have been the subject of a longstanding research tradition (Byrne & Kelley, 1984; Mosher, 1973; Wilson, 1973) which, by and large, functions without reference to the legal complications of obscenity.

Finally, the data utilized in the present chapter are sparse and impressionistic. Not surprisingly, since the production of pornographic films is a crime, access to the pornography industry is extraordinarily difficult to obtain. The present author gained entree to the periphery of the industry, however, as a consequence of his testimony before the Meese Commission (Attorney General's Commission on Pornography, 1986). Meese Commission scientists and pornography actors and actresses were brought together by the Los Angeles media to debate a variety of issues about pornography. Through those debates, I met a number of prominent "stars" (Harry Reems, Kay Parker, etc.), who eventually provided referrals for this research. Thus, besides observing the audition process (at World Wide Modelling), I conducted face-to-face and phone interviews with three very successful pornography actresses (Pat Manning, Kay Parker and Sheri St. Clair) whose combined resumes included performances in over one hundred X-rated films. Additionally, two of these actresses (Pat Manning and Kay Parker) also had considerable experience in the production and promotion of pornography.

Nevertheless, the "data" are obviously problematic. The sample is neither large, random, nor independent, and the assessment technique is biased by comparable systematic error. Despite the consistency of responses among the sample, there was also no external verification of the accuracy of the testimony. Lastly, the author did not observe the production of a pornographic film. Since the production of pornography is a crime, and therefore subject to police intervention, the author concluded that discretion was the better part of valor. As an alternative, however, I was provided access to a documentary film on the production of pornographic movies.

On the other hand, despite all of the obvious limitations inherent in the data, a compelling advantage of this material also exists: it is timely, and it provides suggestions for interventions for a population clearly at risk for the transmission of HIV.

The Pornography Industry in Los Angeles

Five separate entities comprise the pornography industry: agents, talent (actors and actresses), personnel (directors/producers/writers/etc.), financers (production companies/independent financers/etc.), and distributors. Collectively, these entities are a necessary prerequisite to the production of a pornographic movie.

When X-rated movies were produced for theater release, with more substantial budgets, the five separate entities often functioned independently. With the advent of video, however, the entities are less distinct. The cost of producing an X-rated movie has been substantially reduced. Furthermore, a readily accessible marketplace (VCR owners) has now blossomed. Thus, producers, directors, or distributors often finance their own movies, since the cost of production (and the entanglements of distribution) has been diminished.

Although the pornography industry is thriving, the production of a pornographic movie is nonetheless a crime. Pornography is legally deemed "pandering"; i.e., "the crime of inducing a female to become a prostitute." Since pornography actresses are paid for their performances, which usually include explicit sexual sequences, the production of pornography is interpreted as analogous to prostitution. (Interestingly, in light of the illegality of its productions, the industry has attempted to implement a variety of protective "on-location" restrictions to minimize the risk of getting caught. For example, the film location is classified information, and all personnel are required to avoid activities during production that would enhance the risk of prosecution (i.e., drug use, employing underage actors and actresses, etc.).)

Agents act as intermediaries between talent and producers. In Los Angeles, there are two primary agencies for pornography actors and actresses: Jim South's World Wide Modelling and Reb's Pretty Girl. These agencies advertise for nude models in adult-oriented newspapers. Since they are an integral part of the pornography industry, the agencies also receive referrals from inside sources.

Agents interview prospective models, actors and actresses. If deemed marketable and over eighteen years of age, the prospective model, actor, or actress is offered representation by the agency. As part of the commitment for representation, the talent permits the agency to take a nude photograph.

As a first step, the prospective model, actor, or actress is given a list of photographers who specialize in nude modelling. For example, a female model may be hired for a number of still-shoot assignments for adult magazines. These assignments often take five to seven hours, and pay a flat fee of $150–200. If the model is willing to pose with other men or women, however, either simulating or actively engaging in sex, the fee is higher.

A smaller proportion of the talent consents to participation in pornographic movies. Prospective actors and actresses fill out a questionnaire describing the range of activities in which they are willing to engage. This list includes a variety of sexual activities (anal sex, bondage, etc.) and a variety of sexual partners (same sex, Black, Latino, etc.). Although this questionnaire can be updated continuously, it serves the purpose of providing a producer with an a priori range of acceptable activities. This information, incidentally, is critical in an industry which relies upon small production budgets. Since equipment, locations, and personnel are rented or paid per diem, obstacles (such as the need to replace talent) have a costly impact.

Newcomer actors and actresses are usually required to audition for pornographic films. The auditions are often conducted at the agencies, and require the actor or actress to read a short scene, and disrobe. Sexual relations, however, are not an inherent part of auditions.

If an actor or actress is selected for participation in a pornographic film, the agent is paid a flat finder's fee of approximately $55 per day. Thus, unlike the legitimate movie industry where agents assume ten percent of the profits, pornographic agents do not take a percentage of earnings (which for newcomers would be $400-500 per day). It is also true, however, that pornographic agents serve a more limited function, i.e., merely providing the actors' and actress's phone numbers, and assuring that they are over eighteen years of age. Incidentally, it is the latter provision that enhances the agent's liability. For example, in the case of Traci Lord (a sixteen-year-old actress), it was the agent (Jim South) who faced prosecution—even though Traci submitted a bona fide United States passport as proof of age (which, paradoxically, was issued on a false driver's license).

Once an actor or actress becomes popular within the pornography industry, the per-diem salary increases to between $1000 to $1500. In exceptional cases (i.e., Seka), a prominent actress will receive an extraordinary salary ($5000 per diem), plus a percentage of the profits of the movie. Furthermore, a prominent actor or actress can set a maximum limit on the number of sex scenes per day (e.g., two), and require an additional salary for unusual activities (e.g., anal sex). Finally, once talent becomes popular, the agent and auditions become obsolete. Since producers retain the phone numbers of the actors and actresses, contact is made directly. Nevertheless, the agent is still paid the finder's fee.

Actors and actresses who are willing to participate in a wide range of sexual activities, with a variety of sexual partners, enhance their prospects for employment. If the industry, or marketplace, increases the value of a particular activity (e.g., girl/girl scenes, heterosexual anal intercourse), then actors and actresses who consent to this behavior have a greater likelihood of assignments. Refusal to engage in such activities, however, is unlikely to diminish the marketability of a "star." Instead, the sexual activities (anal, girl/girl, etc.) are still filmed, but the scenes are comprised of other actors and actresses. Furthermore, talent with desirable characteristics (very attractive, etc.) also receive continuous employment, despite restrictions on sexual activities. Thus, the prospect for exploitation exists mainly with less marketable (or more impressionable) actors and actresses who enhance their employment by promoting their willingness to engage in unusual activities.

The advent of video has also substantially reduced the length of the production schedule of pornographic films. Typically, such films are budgeted for only a two- to three-day production. Consequently, there is considerable pressure to film scenes in sequence, and to avoid repeated filming of each scene. Furthermore, actors and actresses are expected to arrive promptly, and to have completely memorized their dialogue. On the other hand, production time is specifically allocated to set up sexual sequences. For example, actors and actresses are permitted off-camera time to initiate sexual episodes and become aroused. Moreover, anal intercourse scenes are allocated greater setup time prior to filming. For the most part, pornography actresses exaggerate their sexual arousal, and facilitate insertion with exogenous lubricants (e.g., K-Y jelly).

Once a sexual scene has been set up, it is filmed, usually starting with insertion. The subsequent sexual behaviors or, for that matter, the overall sexual scenes, are determined by a prevailing formula (e.g., "x" number of insertions, "y" number of "cum shoots," "z" number of girl/girl scenes, etc.). This implicit formula also influences the dialogue and direction of pornographic movies.

Once a pornographic movie has been completed, the producer (or production company) usually sells it outright to a distributor. As indicated previously, however, with the advent of video, the distinction between producer and distributor is sometimes clouded, and it is not unusual to have the producer, the director, and the writer all be the same person. Generally, the producer supervises every aspect of production (e.g., obtaining talent, location, financing), whereas the director supervises the lighting, acting, camera angles, and so forth. The writer develops characters, scenes, dialogue and, on rare occasions, plot.

When a film has been purchased for distribution, the distributor makes copies for sale, designs and prints boxes, and initiates promotion of the film. Eventually, the films will be available in retail video stores, or through the mail order market.

Undoubtedly, there are exceptions to this basic structure. Freelance movies are obviously produced, and pornographic "loops"[1] also exist. For the general purpose of suggesting AIDS interventions and research strategies within the pornographic industry, however, this outline represents a reasonable framework.

---

[1] A loop is a type of film used with a small, individual viewer.

AIDS Research and the Pornography Industry

As stated above, pornography actors and actresses engage in the entire repertoire of high-risk sexual behaviors (such as anal intercourse and sex with multiple partners) as a routine requirement of their profession. Since such behaviors undoubtedly enhance the risk of HIV infection and transmission, pornography actors and actresses are an obvious focal point for research.

Pornography actors and actresses are by no means an isolated, homogenous unit. This population overlaps and sexually interacts with other individuals inside (directors, producers, etc.) and outside (boyfriends, girlfriends, spouses, etc.) of the industry. Moreover, the population is not fixed, but instead routinely experiences growth and attrition. Thus, the isolation of a fixed population, for the purpose of this research, was an arbitrary convenience. To compensate for this convenience, however, this population should be conceptualized more broadly to include the relevant individuals (past and present actors and actresses) and their intimate associates. With this caveat in mind, three research objectives seem critical for the pornography population: estimation of the prevalence of HIV, detection of transmission dynamics, and estimation of future HIV infections.

Unfortunately, research objectives are not easily implemented within the pornography industry. Difficulty in gaining access to this population is an obvious obstacle. As indicated above, the production of a pornographic movie is a crime. Thus, the industry is both cliquish and clandestine. Moreover, the pornography industry is not a viable enterprise, but a profitable, "underground" activity.

Nevertheless, the industry is undoubtedly sensitized to AIDS, certainly as a consequence of the recent death of John Holmes.[2] Thus, at the present time, research may be more palatable to the pornography industry — especially if it is conducted with discretion, and does not enhance the industry's criminal or civil liability.

Estimation of the Prevalence of HIV

Paradoxically, the anecdotal reports of prevalence of AIDS within the pornography industry are surprisingly few — especially among heterosexual actors and actresses. If this finding is verifiable, investigation of sero-prevalence (and transmission dynamics) in this group could have considerable relevance to research on heterosexual transmission (Curran et al., 1988; Piot et al., 1988).

The most obvious research strategy within this population is a prospective study of seroconversion of HIV. Initial sampling of HIV would provide a base rate, and subsequent conversion would facilitate knowledge of transmission dynamics. Cooperation from the agents, producer/production companies, and actors and actresses would of course be necessary.

Unfortunately, however, a prospective study is not without limitations. Attenuation of the sample is common — through death, migration, and withdrawal (Kessler and Levin, 1970). Certainly, in the proposed study, sample attrition is a realistic possibility. Par-

---

[2] Holmes, who died of AIDS, was a very prolific actor within the industry. Though used primarily in heterosexual movies, he also participated in homosexual and bisexual films. Moreover, Holmes's drug use has also been raised as a potential source of his infection.

ticipation in pornography is a clandestine activity, usually involving disguised names and appearance (such as dyed hair). Moreover, pornography actors and actresses often spontaneously leave the pornography community in order to assert a different identity in another location. Thus, given the prospect of a nonrandom, nonrepresentative sample to begin with (favoring older and more entrenched actors and actresses), the maintenance of a reasonable and committed population of subjects will take enormous time and effort (MacMahon et al., 1960; Lilienfeld, et al. 1967).

Participation in the study itself will also have a reactive effect upon the sample. Conceivably, the study could enhance the attractiveness of withdrawal from the pornography industry, as a consequence of sensitization to the risk of AIDS. This impact would obviously undermine support for such a project within the industry—especially if it became difficult to maintain or recruit actors and actresses. Alternatively, substantial reductions in the sample size would render statistical treatment of the data meaningless.

Despite the methodological limitations, however, a prospective study of the pornography industry population is still critical, if solely for public health reasons. As stated previously, this population exhibits extraordinary risk for HIV infection. Moreover, pornography actors and actresses mix heterogeneously with the population at large (John Holmes, for instance, was married). Therefore, research of this nature is unquestionably warranted, since it would be relevant to both public health and epidemiologic issues.

Detection of Transmission Dynamics and Estimation of Future HIV Infections

Stochastic models could be introduced to facilitate predictions about the proliferation of HIV within the pornography industry. Such models would permit numerical estimations of significant epidemiological parameters, including probability of infection, length of incubation, and so forth (Abramson & Rothschild, 1988; Anderson, Medley, May & Johnson, 1986; Kaplan, 1988). Statistical tests could also be employed to examine whether hypotheses and observations reliably agree (Bailey, 1975).

For example, Kaplan (1988) has recently introduced a model to determine the prevalence of seropositive individuals and AIDS within a homogenous population, and the conditions under which HIV-infection would remain endemic. As a corollary of this model, Kaplan (1988) examines the situation in which a single HIV-infected person joins an otherwise uninfected population. Since this latter circumstance may have relevance to the pornography industry, Kaplan's model warrants consideration.

Basically, Kaplan examines the probability that a single HIV-infected person will pass the virus to another individual. This model relies upon the expected time for the infected person to infect, the probability of passing the infection, and the rate of finding partners for risky sex (while remaining sexually active). Also of consideration, however, is the fact that the initial infected person will either develop AIDS (with a specific probability), or remain asymptomatic (1 minus the AIDS probability) which, in turn, will determine the individual's duration of sexual activity. For example, if the expected time to infect someone new exceeds the expected time to leave the population (as a consequence of AIDS), Kaplan's model suggests that no epidemic will ensue.

All stochastic models of the proliferation of HIV presume the occurrence of "risky sex." Depending upon the specific definition, this could include unprotected anal or vaginal intercourse. Thus, in either case, pornography actors and actresses warrant inclusion in this category.

There is a quirk in the pornography industry, however, that demands further consideration of the concept of risky sex. For example, in order to verify the authenticity of a male's orgasm, pornography actors customarily ejaculate outside of the vagina, anus, or mouth. Known as "cum shots," these sequences are presumed to be an integral part of the appeal of pornographic films. Therefore, if HIV is transmitted by infected semen (Friedland & Klein, 1987), the risk of transmission may be proportionally lower for pornography actors and actresses. Correspondingly, the assessment of sexual parameters must carefully distinguish the ejaculation site for each sexual sequence.

Where sexual assessment in general is concerned, Abramson (1988) has raised a number of serious issues. Since sexual parameters are critical to the epidemiology of AIDS, then the ultimate efficiency (or utility) of mathematical models is dependent upon the quality and quantity of experimental data on human sexual functioning. Thus, the extent to which sexual variables can be operationalized to permit quantification, as well as the reliability of such data, becomes crucial to determining the relative course of AIDS. And unfortunately, to date, the psychometric saliency of the relevant data on sexual parameters is either marginal or nonexistent. For example, valid measures for such variables as anal intercourse have been difficult to obtain. Therefore, when initiating research with pornography actors and actresses, which ultimately relies upon accurate assessment of sexual information, strict standards of measurement and sampling must be invoked.

Besides Kaplan's (1988) research, there are several other mathematical models (Abramson & Rothschild, 1988; Denning, 1987; May & Anderson, 1987) that would have relevance to this population. In general, these models propose that the selection of sexual partners and the proliferation of HIV depends upon the probability of engaging in high-risk sex (e.g., receptive anal intercourse) times the probability that a selected partner is HIV-positive. And while the absolute number of sexual partners may also be significant (since it is likely to increase the probability of sexual contact with an HIV-positive individual), the critical feature of this "interaction" is the "risk" of the sexual behavior (Abramson & Rothschild, 1988; Kaplan, 1988). For example, Abramson & Rothschild introduce the concept of an "interaction coefficient" which is determined by the "interaction" (which could include sexual intercourse) of various group members (categorized by risk) times the "risk factor" of the behavior between them (which could range from talking to receptive anal intercourse).

Finally, in addition to prospective studies and stochastic models, research within the pornography industry must also examine alternative routes of transmission. Since IV drug use is a critical co-factor for HIV and AIDS (Curran et al, 1988; Friedland & Klein, 1987), drug use within the industry (and with intimate associates) must also be assessed. Although the industry maintains that IV drug use is not evident among actors and actresses (since, as mentioned previously, it would leave traces on their bodies which would be obvious on film, and further jeopardize the viability of the industry), careful measurement of such behavior is important. Also, if "cum shots" lower the risks of HIV infection for pornography actors and actresses, research should examine the differential rates of semen-transmitted STDs (Sexually Transmitted Diseases). (HIV, gonorrhea, etc.) and contact-transmitted STDs (genital herpes, condyloma) (Harris & Abramson, 1988; Houck & Abramson, 1986), using groups matched for risk (i.e., pornography actors and actresses contrasted with prostitutes or Gay bathhouse patrons).

AIDS Intervention Within the Pornography Industry

There are two primary objectives for intervention within the pornography industry: to enhance knowledge about the risks and transmission of HIV, and to make safe sex an integral part of pornographic films.

Cooperation from the industry is an obvious prerequisite for achieving these objectives. Certainly, in order to effectuate a permanent intervention, the industry must be amenable to change, and take responsibility for the advocacy of safe sex.

At present, there is evidence to suggest that the industry is making at least a token effort to institute behavioral change within pornographic films. A number of films utilizing safe sex have been produced (such as the sequels to "Behind the Green Door" and "Deep Insider Trading"), and a number of production companies, among them Platnum Productions, are attempting to incorporate safe sex within their repertoire of sexual sequences. Finally, at least one production company (Catalina) incorporates a safe-sex promotional clip as an introduction to every film.

Pornography actresses are also being more cautious about the risks of transmitting HIV. Seka, a prominent actress within the industry, required HIV antibody tests for all actors and actresses in one of her recent movies. Unfortunately, the prospect of an HIV infectious latency period (Lui, et al, 1986; Medley et al, 1987) compromises the efficacy of this approach. Viable alternatives, however, exist. The pervasive impact of public forums, such as press conferences, are capable of influencing the pornography industry. For example, Nina Hartley (a prominent pornography actress) was recently televised advocating safe sex. In this circumstance, the effectiveness of her appeal within the industry can be assessed by measuring the degree of adherence to safe sex practices in her subsequent movies.

On the other hand, if media coverage increases public recognition of HIV transmission within the pornography industry, such exposure may also generate renewed efforts toward prosecution. Like Gay bathhouses, the pornography industry may ultimately be targeted as a public health hazard. There is considerable debate within the public health literature (Richwald, et al, 1988), however, about whether this strategy facilitates or minimizes public health initiatives.

Therefore, in order to initiate effective prevention strategies within the industry, all entities must be cooperative. For example, agents could require evidence of continuous antibody status as a prerequisite of employment. While such a requirement may engender ethical and legal complications (Dickens, 1988; Walters, 1988), the necessity of engaging in risky sexual behavior as a consequence of one's profession may require some unusual accommodations. Certainly, such testing should be voluntary and recorded solely by alias, that is without reference to the actor or actress's real name.

Unfortunately, the prospect of gaining cooperation—and funding—for continuous ELISA or Western Blot tests from pornographic agents is relatively slim. As indicated previously, such agencies function merely as clearinghouses for potential talent. Furthermore, agents become obsolete when actors and actresses gain prominence. Perhaps if agents were deemed liable for the antibody status of prospective actors and actresses, greater cooperation could be obtained. Civil liability in such cases, however, is a complex, and unresolved issue (Dickens, 1988; Girardi, Keese, Traver & Cooksey, 1988).

Similarly, production entities (e.g., producers, production companies, financiers, and distributors) do not have reputations for magnanimity. Although some companies have obviously initiated safe-sex films, such circumstances are the exception rather than the rule. Generally, except for stars, most pornography actors and actresses are deemed expendable or, at best, exchangeable. Moreover, the continuous search for new faces mediates commitment to the rank and file. Finally, production entities tend to emphasize profit, rather than commitment to talent. If industry revenues are reduced because of fear of AIDS, however, production will presumably exhibit more AIDS consciousness.

Consequently, pornography actors and actresses represent the most effective means for initiating AIDS intervention in the industry. Since the industry is dependent upon the profitable marketing of stars, such individuals are capable of leveraging safe-sex changes. Obviously, actors and actresses carry the greatest burden of risk for AIDS within the industry. Therefore, the advantages for change, and the prospects for advocacy, rest with such individuals.

Targeting pornography stars is the most direct means of implementing change. Such stars should be thoroughly trained in AIDS prevention, and encouraged to require safe sex in all films. Safe sex should include condoms, spermicides, and the avoidance of ejaculation within the mouth, vagina, or rectum. Also, extensive set-up time should be initiated for all sexual sequences, to minimize lesions during insertion. Similarly, the sexual sequences themselves should be designed to avoid trauma to the vagina or rectum. Finally, to facilitate attraction (within the industry) to safe sex sequences, suggestions should be made to enhance the eroticism, or humor, of safe sex encounters.

Since several prominent actors and actresses are independently initiating significant changes, efforts at AIDS prevention could attempt to more formally organize such individuals. Unlike the mainstream film industry, which has the Screen Actors Guild, the pornography industry is devoid of unionized groups. The collective effort of influential stars, however, would obviously facilitate rapid modifications. Furthermore, collective efforts, initiated by past and present stars, could be more persuasive in attracting the unconvinced (i.e., the young, the "invincible," etc.) to their ranks. Finally, although such efforts will undoubtably fail to incorporate all members of the pornography profession, if a sizeable group were assembled the industry would obviously take notice.

As indicated in the introduction of this chapter, the strategies in this chapter are being offered without reference to the legal status of pornography. One could argue, however, that since pornography is a crime, and since pornography actors and actresses are at risk for AIDS, the most efficient solution would be to shut down the industry. Unfortunately, even if this solution were viable, the prospects of immediately shutting down the industry are minuscule. Thus, like prostitution the pornography industry seems to prevail. And as such, given its durability, the pornography industry warrants prevention for itself, and the community at large. Furthermore, if the American populace becomes more conscientious (and restrictive) about sexuality, pornography may actually increase in appeal as a "fantasy" alternative. Therefore, since a sizeable portion of the American populace already rents pornographic videos, the incorporation of safe sex sequences could enhance attitudes and behavior about safe sex.

Conclusion

This chapter introduced the issues relevant to AIDS and the pornography industry. Given the prevalence of high-risk behaviors, and the recent example of the late John Holmes, pornography actors and actresses represent a critical population for study. Consequently, the research strategies and educational interventions proposed here warrant close consideration.

References

1. Abramson, P.R. (1988). "Sexual Assessment and the Epidemiology of AIDS." *Journal of Sex Research*, 25, in press.
2. Abramson, P.R. & Hayashi, H. (1984). "Pornography in Japan: Cross-Cultural and Theoretical Considerations." In N. M. Malamuth and E. Donnerstein (Eds.) *Pornography and Sexual Aggression*. New York: Academic Press.
3. Abramson, P.R. & Rothschild, B. (1988). "Sex, Drugs and Matrices: Mathematical Prediction of HIV Infection." *Journal of Sex Research*, 25, 106–122.
4. Anderson, R.M., Medley, G.F., May, R.M., & Johnson, A.M. (1986). "A Preliminary Study of the Transmission Dynamics of the Human Immunodeficiency Virus (HIV), the Causative Agent of AIDS." *IMA Journal of Mathematics Applied in Medicine & Biology*, 3, 229–263.
5. Attorney General's Commission on Pornography (1986). Final Report. U.S. Government Printing Office.
6. Bailey, N.T.J. (1975). *The Mathematical Theory of Infectious Diseases*. London: Charles Griffin & Co.
7. Baldwin, J.D. & Baldwin, J.I. (1988). "Factors Affecting AIDS-Related Sexual Risk-Taking Behavior Among College Students." *Journal of Sex Research*, 25, 181–196.
8. Byrne, D. & Kelley, K. (1984). "Pornography and Sex Research." In N.M. Malamuth and E. Donnerstein (Eds.) *Pornography and Sexual Aggression*. New York: Academic Press.
9. Curran, J.W., Jaffe, H.W., Hardy, A.M., Morgan, W.M., Selik, R.M., & Dondero, T.J. (1988). "Epidemiology of HIV Infection and AIDS in the United States." *Science*, 239, 610–616.
10. Dickens, B.M. (1988). "Legal Rights and Duties in the AIDS Epidemic." *Science*, 239, 580–586.
11. Fineberg, H.V. (1988). "Education to Prevent AIDS: Prospects and Obstacles." *Science*, 239, 592–596.
12. Friedland, G.H. & Klein, R. (1987). "Transmission of the Human Immunodeficiency Virus." *The New England Journal of Medicine*, 317, 1125–1135.
13. Girardi, J.A., Keese, R.M., Traver, L.B., & Cooksey, D.R. (1988). "Psychotherapist Responsibility in Notifying Individuals at Risk for Exposure to HIV." *Journal of Sex Research*, 25, 1–27.
14. Grant, R. M., Wiley, J.A. & Winkelstein, W. (1987). "Infectivity of the Human Immunodeficiency Virus: Estimates from a Prospective Study of Homosexual Men." *Journal of Infectious Disease*, 156, 189–193.
15. Harris, G. N. & Abramson, P.R. (1988). "Personality Correlates of the Clinical Sequelae of Genital Herpes." *Journal of Research in Personality*, in press.
16. Houck, E.L. & Abramson, P.R. (1986). "Masturbatory Guilt and the Psychological Consequences of Sexually Transmitted Diseases Among Women." *Journal of Research in Personality*, 20, 267–275.

17. Kaplan, E.H. (1988). "What Are the Risks of Risky Sex? Powerful Insights from Simple Models." Under editorial review.
18. Kessler, I.I. & Levin, M.L. (1970). *The Community as an Epidemiologic Laboratory.* Baltimore: The Johns Hpokins Press.
19. Kingsley, L.A., Kaslow, R., Rinaldo, C.R., Detrie, K., Odaka, N., VanRaden, M., Detels, R., Polk, B.F., Chmiel, J., Kelsey, S.F., Ostrow, D., Vissher, B. (1987). "Risk Factors for Seroconversion to Human Immunodeficiency Virus Among Male Homosexuals." *Lancet,* February 14th, 345–348.
20. Lilienfeld, A.M., Pedersen, E. & Dowd, J.E. (1967). *Cancer Epidemiology: Methods of Study.* Baltimore: The Johns Hopkins Press.
21. Lui, K, Lawrence, D.N., Morgan, W.M., Peterman, T.A., Haverkos, H.W. & Bregman, D.J. (1986). "A Model-Based Approach for Estimating the Mean Incubation Period of Transfusion-Associated Acquired Immunodeficiency Syndrome." Proceedings of the National Academy of Sciences, 83, 3051–3055.
22. MacMahon, B., Pugh, T.F. & Ipsen, J. (1960). *Epidemiologic Methods.* Boston: Little, Brown & Company.
23. Malamuth, N.M. & Donnerstein, E. (Eds.) (1984). *Pornography and Sexual Aggression.* New York: Academic Press.
24. May, R.M. & Anderson, R.M. (1987). "Transmission Dynamics of HIV Infection." *Nature,* 326, 137–142.
25. Medley, G.F., Anderson, R.M., Cox, D.R., & Billard, L. (1987). "Incubation Period of AIDS in Patients Infected Via Blood Transfusion." *Nature,* 328, 719–721.
26. Mosher, D.L. (1973). "Sex Differences, Sex Experience, Sex Guilt and Explicitly Sexual Films." *Journal of Social Issues,* 29, 95–112.
27. McKusic, L.M., Horstman, W., & Coates, T.J. (1985). "Aids and Sexual Behavior Reported by Gay Men in San Francisco." *American Journal of Public Health,* 75, 493–496.
28. Osborn, J. E. (1986a). "The AIDS Epidemic: An Overview of the Science." *Issues in Science and Technology,* Winter, 40–55.
29. Osborn, J.E. (1986b). "The AIDS Epidemic: Multidisciplinary Trouble." *The New England Journal of Medicine,* 314, 779–782.
30. Parker, R. (19??). "Acquired Immunodeficiency Syndrome in Urban Brazil." Medical Anthropology Quarterly, 155–175.
31. Penrod, S. & Linz, D. (1984). "Using Psychological Research on Violent Pornography to Inform Legal Change." In N.M. Malamuth and E. Donnerstein (Eds.). *Pornography and Sexual Aggression.* New York: Academic Press.
32. Piot, P., Plummer, F.A., Mhalu, F.S., Lamboray, J., Chin, J. & Mann, J.M. (1988). "AIDS: An International Perspective." *Science,* 239, 573–579.
33. Richards, D.A.J. (1974-1975). "Free Speech and Obscenity Law: Toward a Moral Theory of the First Amendment." *University of Pennsylvania Law Review,* 123, 45–91.
34. Richards, D.A.J. (1979). "Commercial Sex and the Rights of the Person: A Moral Argument for the Decriminalization of Prostitution." *University of Pennsylvania Law Review,* 127, 1195–1287.

35. Richards, D.A.J. (1982). *Sex, Drugs, Death, and the Law*. Totowa, New Jersey: Rowman & Littlefield.
36. Richwald, G.A., Morisky, D.E., Kyle, G.R., Kristal, A.R., Gerber, M.M., & Friedland, J.M. (1988). "Sexual Activities in Bathhouses in Los Angeles County: Implications for AIDS Prevention Education." *Journal of Sex Research,* 25, 169–180.
37. Technical Report of the Commission on Obscenity and Pornography (1971). "The Marketplace: The Industry." Volume 3, U.S. Government Printing Office.
38. Walters, L. (1988). "Ethical Issues in the Prevention and Treatment of HIV Infection and AIDS." *Science,* 239, 597–603.
39. Wilson, W.C. (1973). "Pornography: The Emergence of a Social Issue and the Beginning of Psychological Study." *Journal of Social Issues,* 29, 7–17.

Chapter 3

Looking Back and Forward: Hospital Responses to Epidemics and AIDS

Robin Lloyd

WITH AIDS FINALLY recognized as a social, as well as medical, issue in the United States, many policy-makers are turning their attention to how hospitals treat AIDS patients. This chapter explores the impact of AIDS and of previous epidemics on hospital health care.

Comparing hospital responses to AIDS with those of past epidemics, it is clear that we needn't discuss AIDS as though we've never encountered anything like it before. At least in the United States, AIDS poses to the 1980s hospital many of the same challenges that were faced by health care workers in the past. For this reason, it is crucial that researchers and policy-makers be aware of the history of American experiences with such diseases as cholera, tuberculosis, and venereal disease.

This chapter begins by examining the features of previous epidemics that influence how hospitals are responding to AIDS today. It then looks at hospital responses to AIDS in detail, focusing attention not only on financial variables, but also on organizational, attitudinal and ethical issues. Finally, it concludes with recommendations for future research and policy on hospitals and AIDS.

Historical Examples

Historians of hospitals (Rosenberg,1987; Rosner,1982; Starr,1982) and epidemics (Brandt,1987; Rosenberg,1962; Dubos and Dubos,1952) offer analyses that are a useful context in which to view the link between the goals and principles of hospital care. Hospital responses to cholera, tuberculosis, and venereal disease are distinguishable from one another by their reactive, versus proactive, characters, their efforts to prevent versus efforts to cure, and their different organizational settings.

The first hospitals in the United States refused to admit contagious, chronic, and incurable patients, partly in an effort to protect their staff (Rosenberg,1987). There was perhaps legitimate concern about triggering an epidemic within hospitals (Rosenberg, 1987). Victims of epidemics, therefore, were unlikely to be admitted to hospitals. Early nineteenth century hospitals also made a practice of judging the moral worthiness of potential admissions. Smallpox and cholera victims, for example, were widely stigmatized.

The earliest, small hospitals of the nineteenth century would close when an epidemic began spreading through the institution. As hospitals grew larger, however, closure became impractical. Instead, hospitals implemented procedures for dealing with patients thought to be spreading epidemic diseases like influenza or childbed fever. Once located, such patients were isolated in wards or rooms, and their former dwellings were fumigated, white-washed, scoured, aired, and emptied of infected linens.

Well-administered hospitals tried to prevent the spread of epidemics by such measures as avoiding crowding, enforcing cleanliness, ensuring ventilation, changing linens, emptying bedpans frequently, removing uneaten food quickly, installing smooth-surfaced floors for easy cleaning, and installing efficient sewers and drains to prevent the buildup of poisons (Rosenberg,1987).

Even with advances in medicine and the growth in their acceptance by the general public, hospitals still concentrated on acute and curable patients (Rosenberg,1987). For example, since medical treatment was of little use, hospitals were generally unwilling to admit tubercular patients. Even when hospitals became centers for teaching medicine, admissions changed very little. Tuberculosis patients, for instance, were admitted only when they were useful for classroom purposes (Rosenberg,1987).

In the latter half of the nineteenth century, urban hospitals began to provide special services for patients with specific diseases, including those linked to epidemics. For instance, New York's hospitals in the 1880s included a chronic disease hospital, a smallpox hospital, a fever hospital, and units for incurables and epileptics (Rosenberg,1987). Nevertheless, it is still true today that hospitals admit patients primarily during the peak of serious disease, and strongly prefer patients who have diseases with known cures and proven treatments (Starr,1982).

Cholera

Historically, "ad hoc" hospitals have been responsible for dealing with outbreaks of incurable illnesses. During the three U.S. cholera epidemics of the nineteenth century, for instance, temporary hospitals were created within days (Rosenberg, 1962). In 1832, shortly after the city's first cholera cases were reported, the New York Board of Health organized four hospitals: in the Hall of Records, a school, an old bank, and an abandoned work shed.

This is not to say that hospital care was, by today's standards, even remotely satisfactory. During the second U.S. cholera epidemic in 1849, hospitals for the disease were poorly staffed by volunteer nurses and doctors and lacked sufficient funds (Rosenberg,1962). Most patients at these hospitals lay nearly dead, with dirty sheets their only bedclothes. Not surprisingly, even physicians at these hospitals wanted them closed.

Medical practitioners were more successful with the final cholera epidemic, in 1866. Public health officials combined home visits with quarantines and improvement of sanitary conditions in housing and urban areas. (Rosenberg,1962). In other words, hospital care for the treatment of cholera patients was largely abandoned, once it was discovered that effective treatment of the epidemic depended on a change in the lifestyles of entire urban populations (Rosenberg,1962).

The strengthening of public health practices in 1866 proved to be the key to halting cholera's spread. Upon the very first cholera death in New York, the Board of Health implemented a plan that included reporting cases to the local police station, telegraphing the news to the health board, and dispatching men to disinfect the sick person's premises within an hour. Even before the first reported cholera case, vials of medications (of dubious effectiveness) were distributed to poor people who complained of cholera's early symptoms. Most American cities, however, lacked a board of health like New York's, and their high cholera death counts reflected their lack of organization (Rosenberg,1962). In the case of New York, Rosenberg succinctly argues, physicians discovered that their effective role in treating cholera was not to find a cure, but to prevent cholera transmission (1962).

Rosenberg (1962) also points out that medicine's initial failure in the prevention and treatment of cholera catalyzed a complete overhaul of the field of medicine. Experience showed that cholera patients did best when they were simply kept warm and given no medication other than broth or wine. Medical practitioners no longer asked whether a remedy was effective in treating a disease; rather, they learned to ask how best to alleviate the symptoms (Rosenberg,1962). Thus, hospital, medical, and public health responses to cholera achieved success once they assumed a proactive, rather than reactive, stance. In the first two cholera epidemics, while health care officials responded quickly, the responses included little advanced planning. In anticipation of the third epidemic, however, public health officials tried to *halt the spread* of, rather than try to cure people of, the disease.

The proactive response included the coordinated efforts of several public institutions experienced in dealing with cholera. Thus, hospital health care was less important in containing the spread of cholera than was a coordinated effort from the community and public health system. Clearly, hospitals alone were not responsible for the successful treatment of cholera; instead, the organizational form of effective cholera treatment was multidimensional and centered in the community.

Tuberculosis

As with cholera, hospital treatment offered no cure for tuberculosis, and efforts to halt the disease were initially reactive. Tuberculosis patients were systematically excluded from hospitals in the nineteenth century (Rosenberg,1987). According to Dubos and Dubos (1952), questions about the transmission, treatment and underlying causes of tuberculosis puzzled public health officials and medical practitioners well into the twentieth century.

Rosenberg and Dubos and Dubos describe the emergence, and epidemiological success, of sanitoria in controlling tuberculosis. Around the turn of the century, unlike conventional hospital objectives for the treatment of infectious diseases, sanitoria were created to serve as havens for the recovery of patients, quarantine infectious patients from the general public, and educate patients about the spread of tuberculosis (Dubos and Dubos, 1952).

The sanitorium movement began in eighteenth century Europe. In the United States, however, the apparent effectiveness of sanitoria was "discovered" independently in the nineteenth century by a man with tuberculosis who spent time in the Adirondacks and noticed improvement in his health. Fresh air and relaxation were given the credit, and soon stays in sanitoria became quite common (Dubos and Dubos,1952). An institutional solution to controlling tuberculosis was devised, therefore, by a lay person with tuberculosis.

As with cholera, success in controlling tuberculosis had little to do with a cure; rather, it rested on efforts to prevent transmission. Again, the general hospital did not prove to be the appropriate organizational form for the treatment and control of tuberculosis.

Venereal Disease

Like cholera and tuberculosis, venereal disease has challenged — and helped transform — conventional medicine and health care. With venereal disease, health care was broadened to include psychosocial and educational (as well as clinical) tasks (Brandt, 1987). Due to the stigma attached to venereal disease, some physicians chose not to treat patients. Others specialized in VD treatment despite their own stigmatization as "clap doctors." Facilities for the treatment of VD, however, were not created until decades after the spread of the disease reached epidemic proportions (Brandt, 1987). Many hospitals, using the criteria of deservedness, refused to admit or treat patients well into the end of the nineteenth century: individuals carrying venereal disease were often seen as "not deserving," and were denied medical treatment.

In the early twentieth century, cities with strong public health boards introduced VD clinics. During World War I, the military established prophylactic stations to combat venereal disease among soldiers (Brandt,1987). However, many infected soldiers chose not to visit the stations because of long lines and the derision to which they were subjected while waiting for treatment. While military health officials recognized that treatment, not education, curbed the spread of venereal disease among the ranks, they remained uncomfortable with the notion that providing prophylaxis for venereal disease was akin to promoting licentious sexual activity. As a result, efforts to curb VD remained uncoordinated and only marginally effective throughout the War (Brandt, 1987).

Following World War I, venereal disease spread even more rapidly and the federal government implemented stronger methods to halt its transmission. Rather than treating those infected, however, the government blamed prostitutes for its spread. Between 1918 and 1920, some 18,000 women were held in detention houses (Brandt, 1987). Needless to say, this effort did not successfully halt the spread of venereal diseases.

Hospitals, and alternative institutions set up by ambivalent administrators, remained largely unsuccessful. Without questioning medical practices and assumptions about human behavior, the campaign to halt venereal disease was ineffective, especially relative to the success of cholera hospitals and tuberculosis sanitoria. In the case of venereal disease, federal, local, and military responses remained cure-centered and reactive, rather than proactive. Neither hospitals nor alternatively organized clinics and prophylactic stations provided an effective organizational response to VD epidemics.

Hospital Responses to AIDS

Several lessons about controlling epidemics can be drawn from the historical examples of cholera, tuberculosis, and venereal disease. First, proactive approaches in cooperation with patients and their communities apparently produce results. Second, disease-specific hospitals seem more effective than general hospitals. Third, the best treatments include not only medical but educational and psychosocial components. These conclusions must be the cornerstone of any examination of today's hospital responses to AIDS.

While hospitals recognize the Centers for Disease Control's (CDC) guidelines for preventing transmission of the HIV from patients to others (CDC, 1987, 1985), little information exists on their enactment of those guidelines. Some physicians and journalists have explored the practical concerns of medical professionals (Steinbrook, Lo, Tirpack, Dilley and Volberding,1985; Wachter,1986), but rarely do they focus on the role of hospitals in responding to AIDS. When they do—as in the case of Adrulis, Beers, Bentley, Gage, Link, Feinbold, Charap, Freeman and Shelov—they tend to address AIDS only as an economic challenge. While economic concerns are certainly important, there are several additional variables that should be of equal consideration. Few researchers, for instance, look for ways that AIDS is changing medical and hospital organization, attitudes, and behaviors of health care workers and patients, and the goals and purview of conventional medicine in the AIDS crisis. What follows is gleaned from the limited sources available, and presents a research agenda for hospital response to AIDS.

Finances

Hospitals are unable to foot the bill for the average stay of a patient with AIDS (*Hospitals,* January 5, 1986; *American Medical News,* November 15, 1985). Most researchers agree with the 1985 CDC estimate that costs for treating AIDS patients are double those for treating all other patients (Bloom and Carliner, 1988). More specifically, the CDC estimates that the average stay for an AIDS patient is $830 per day (*Hospitals,* January 5, 1986), much higher than the per-day charges for patients with other infectious diseases. A number of researchers concur; their estimates range from $683 per day to $1003 per day (Bloom and Carliner, 1988). The results of two studies (Landesman, Ginzburg, and Weiss, 1985; Seage, Landers, Barry, Groopman, Lamb, and Epstein, 1986) estimate the current lifetime cost of treating an AIDS patient at about $45,000. Other researchers

There are a variety of reasons for the higher cost of treating AIDS. AIDS patients staying in Intensive Care Units (ICUs) incur much higher fees and have longer hospital stays (Scitovsky, Cline, and Lee, 1986; *American Medical News,* November 15, 1986). AIDS patients require multiple hospitalizations during the course of their illness (Benfer, 1987). There are higher rates of homelessness among IV drug users who become AIDS patients, and this leads to longer hospital stays (*Hospitals,* January 5, 1986; Scitovsky et al., 1986). AIDS patients who are immuno-compromised with symptoms of fever, shortness of breath, headaches, and confusion require exhaustive and often invasive procedures to keep them from getting sicker (Wachter, 1986). AIDS patients with lymphadenopathy require more costly immunologic evaluations, screening for infections, and lymph node biopsies (Groopman and Detsky, 1983), and AIDS patients require additional laboratory work, more pharmacy and professional fees, and more supplies, therapy and X-rays (Seage et al., 1986). Supply costs rise, especially when hospitals adhere to universal precautions (Benfer, 1987). In addition, AIDS patients may incur substantial costs for social services (*Hospitals,* January 5, 1986).

Given this context, it is clear that some changes will have to be made in order to avoid a financial catastrophe for hospitals. Some commentators offer recommendations for dealing with the financial costs of AIDS (*American Medical News,* Nov. 15, 1985; Groopman and Detsky, 1983). For example, Groopman and Detsky (1983) suggest that certain hospitals be designated as centers for AIDS treatment, and that funding be coordinated between government and the private sector for optimal support of AIDS research (1983). A more recent article reports that hospitals have started financial planning for the treatment of AIDS patients (*American Medical News,* November 15, 1985). Physicians and hospital administrators advocate changes in Medicare eligibility that will allow greater reimbursements for the treatment of AIDS patients (Benfer, 1987; *American Medical News,* Nov. 15, 1985).

Hospital organization

Some hospitals are changing their structural organization in response to the numbers and needs of AIDS patients (e.g., Benfer, 1987; *Hospitals,* January 5, 1986). Paralleling their responses to previous epidemics such as smallpox, some hospitals now specialize in AIDS health care while others deal with AIDS patients simply by isolating them and treating them as any other infectious patient. Still other hospitals have no formal programs for AIDS, for fear that the label "AIDS hospital" will reduce their patient base (Nary, 1987). Stigma has always followed patients with epidemic diseases (especially those acquired through sexual contact) and the medical staff who take care of them.

Despite the potential for stigmatization, San Francisco General Hospital has instituted both an inpatient unit and an outpatient clinic for people with AIDS (Wachter, 1986). As a resident at this hospital, Wachter comments that these special units, plus community response, have greatly enhanced the care received by people with AIDS. Wachter speculates that better care translates into a reduced length of inpatient stays — from what might take fifty days in New York to less than twenty-two days in San Francisco. Other features of the San Francisco General hospital model include private rooms for dying patients, outpatient counseling for patients newly diagnosed with AIDS, patient support groups, a twenty-four-hour telephone hotline for AIDS questions, physician referrals, and educational programs (*American Medical News,* January 10, 1986).

The relative success of the San Francisco General Hospital model harks back to previous hospital successes with epidemics. The proactive, disease-specific, and community-coordinated features of San Francisco General's response are similar to those that prevented the spread of cholera in 1866. Rather than rely simply on education (as with venereal disease during World War I), or simply on reactive clinical treatment (as with the earlier cholera epidemic of 1832), San Francisco General integrates a variety of medical and non-medical treatments.

Other hospitals (such as Johns Hopkins and Henry Ford Hospitals) have instituted special wards or sections for the treatment of AIDS patients, or have dedicated the entire institution as a center for AIDS treatment (such as Charity Hospital in New Orleans). Recently established New York State Health Department regulations encourage hospitals that become centers for treating AIDS patients to emphasize home care, hospice care, outpatient clinic services, and counseling services (*American Medical News,* February 14, 1986). Green et al. (1987) claim that many hospitals treat people with AIDS as outpatients for problems that would normally have been treated on an inpatient basis.

Thus, conventional functions of hospitals are shifting as it becomes obvious that standard organizational practices can accommodate neither the numbers of AIDS patients in high incidence regions nor the extra labor they require. Similarly, public health officials report that AIDS units result in more efficient care, which will reduce inpatient costs and help quell the public's fears of infection (*Hospitals,* January 5, 1986). In the past, tuberculosis sanitoria were created as a better response to patient needs. Similarly, AIDS hospitals may find that changes in conventional medical and hospital practices may better serve not only patients, but also staff, administrators, and the community.

Physicians currently agree that AIDS units might allow better coordination of inpatient services, improve follow-up of patients, more efficiently use social services, and increase knowledge about AIDS treatment (Landesman, Ginzburg, and Weiss, 1985). One physician does warn that AIDS patients in such units might be subject to stigmatization and therefore receive inferior care (1985, p. 524). Since Wachter's (1986) later experience, however, counters Landesman, Ginzburg, and Weiss's expectations, there is evidence that the positives of AIDS units outweigh any negatives.

The issue of quarantining and/or treating in isolation patients with epidemic diseases remains unresolved. Today, not all hospitals choose to isolate AIDS patients. For instance, St. Luke's-Roosevelt Hospital Center in New York distributes AIDS patients across units so that additional nursing staff need not be hired (*Hospitals,* January 5, 1986). Administrators at a Houston hospital claim also that AIDS admissions have not necessitated any organizational changes, and that AIDS patients are treated like any other patient with an infectious disease (*Hospitals,* January 5, 1986).

Future research should look for other ways in which hospitals are responding to AIDS patients' needs for extra care. Are more nurses being hired? Are there work "speed-ups?" Are patients being short-changed in the care they require?

Wachter (1986) suggests there should be a change in the use of already existing hospital units. Noting an eighty-seven percent mortality figure of patients admitted to San Francisco General's Intensive Care Unit, Wachter argues for more frank discussion between patients and physicians about hospital and non-hospital alternatives to ICU care. In light of the lack of effective ICU therapies for AIDS patients, Wachter discourages admitting AIDS patients to these units. Dialogue between patients and physicians is crucial. Less emphasis on drug therapies and more on prevention and changing lifestyles may bring the same successes as those eventually achieved with cholera and venereal disease.

Wachter and others (such as Volberding in *American Medical News*, Oct. 18, 1985) claim that AIDS is changing the very ways in which medicine is performed. Wachter's discussion of ICU use suggests that AIDS, like cholera and tuberculosis, may change the conventions of patient treatment in hospitals. These changes may persist over time and affect all patients, not just those with AIDS. For instance, physicians may alter ICU admissions policies. Earlier home discharges may be encouraged for patients with incurable, debilitating diseases. Future research is necessary to investigate other long-term organizational changes in hospitals attributable to AIDS.

Discharge planning

Hospitals cannot discharge AIDS patients until adequate care and shelter are arranged. This requirement is problematic for several reasons. First, AIDS patients who are intravenous drug users are often homeless (*Hospitals,* January 5, 1986). Second, many nursing homes that care for discharged patients with chronic and fatal diseases are refusing to admit people with AIDS. (*AIDS Alert,* January, 1987). Third, even patients who enter the hospital with homes and sufficient funds, upon discharge often no longer can afford to pay rent or fees for care. (*Hospitals,* January 5, 1986).

One public health official predicts that nursing homes will warm to the idea of admitting AIDS patients when administrators recognize that there is money to be made by competing with hospitals for long-term care beds (*AIDS Alert,* 1987). Another promising prospect is that health departments in some states are modifying Medicaid eligibility to facilitate higher reimbursements for AIDS patient care in nursing homes (*AIDS Alert,* January, 1987). This effort has been effective in raising AIDS admissions in at least one nursing home in the state of Maryland.

Nursing homes, however, may not be able to meet the care needs of all AIDS patients. AIDS patients require far more emotional support and direct nursing care than is conventionally provided by such homes (Green, et al., 1987). While there are some alternatives to nursing homes, such as hospices and home care, Medicaid coverage for these services is often not available (*Hospitals,* January 5, 1986). Hospital administrators acknowledge that creative planning for post-hospital care of AIDS patients is crucial. Alternatives—such as the rooming house for homeless AIDS patients provided by the Shanti project in San Francisco—must be recognized by hospital administrators, so that more care alternatives can be created.

Staff attitudes and behavior

Unlike most of today's infectious diseases, AIDS is at least fifty-five percent fatal and has no known cure or truly effective treatment. This feature of AIDS frightens many health care workers (*AIDS Alert,* October 1, 1986). While health care workers have always risked contact with infectious diseases, their fears have often been quelled by their awareness of cures, vaccines, or treatments. For instance, nurses frequently contract hepatitis from their patients, but hospitals usually successfully treat both hepatitis A and B. In contrast, health workers know there is currently no medically established "fix" for

AIDS. The intense labor of treating people with AIDs, combined with patients' high hospital mortality, may also reduce morale among health care workers.

A study of pediatric and medical residents (Link et al.,1988) reports that residents have moderate to major concerns about acquiring AIDS from their patients. The report's data is drawn from responses to a questionnaire completed by 250 residents staffing seven New York City hospitals. Concern was higher among less experienced residents, among residents who had treated larger numbers of AIDS patients, and among medical rather than pediatric residents. Concern did not depend upon physicians' frequency of splash or needle-stick exposures to the AIDS virus.

One fourth of the surveyed physicians would choose not to continue to care for AIDS patients if given a choice. On the other hand, the residents reported little resentment about having to care for AIDS patients. As the authors of the study indicate, the results of the questionnaire are "disquieting," and point to a great need for research on the relationship between attitudes and behaviors of health care workers dealing with AIDS.

Link and his colleagues recommend that house staff create formal education programs and provide personal counseling for health care workers (1988). Future studies of this kind might survey health care workers other than residents, and workers located in regions other than New York. The survey instrument might include questions probing behavioral, as well as attitudinal, changes health care workers claim to have made since dealing with AIDS. Such data might fruitfully be compared to data collected from a similar population of health care workers with little or no experience with AIDS. In addition, direct observation would enhance any survey research on hospital staffs' responses to AIDS.

Responsibility and refusal to treat

Clearly, no hospital can operate without the cooperation of its staff. While the Hippocratic oath and legal codes for health care remain intact (Banks, 1987), in practice there is ambiguity surrounding hospital and physician responsibilities and rights in the treatment of patients with AIDS. Many authors and reporters have documented refusals by physicians, nurses, and paramedics to treat AIDS patients (see *American Medical News,* November 8, 1985; Banks, 1987; Loewy, 1986). The media describe many instances of discrimination by health care workers (Ponsford, 1987; *Washington Post National Weekly,* December 8, 1986; *New York Times,* June 2, 1985; Steinbrook, 1985). In a sense, little has changed since the nineteenth century.

Yet, many physicians, and the Surgeon General, argue that health care workers have an obligation to treat AIDS patients and assume some degree of risk, much as they have with other diseases (Kim and Perfect, 1988; Hospitals, December 5, 1987; Loewy, 1986; Conte et al., 1983). One physician (Frank, 1986) argues that health care professionals are trained to take life-threatening risks, just like fire fighters who must risk their lives to put out a fire. He admits that AIDS frightens health care workers because it has no known cure. Still, he argues, the profession's integrity must be maintained and physicians have a responsibility to treat AIDS patients.

In hospital settings, even health care workers with good intentions report more intensely emotional responses to treating AIDS patients than in treating other patients (*Hospitals,* January 5, 1986; Steinbrook, 1985; Wachter, 1986). Some physicians (Wachter, Luce, Turner, Volberding, and Hopewell, 1986) who recognize the virtual death sentence of ICU admissions express frustration following treatment discussions with patients. Watching so many young, previously healthy patients die is challenging even for experienced health care professionals (Wachter, 1986). Steinbrook et al. (1985) report a colleague's description of talking about life-sustaining treatments with an AIDS patient to be like "telling your brother he is going to die."

Matters are further complicated by emotionally-charged conflicts between house staff and sub-specialty physicians about proper treatment of AIDS patients (Wachter, 1986; Steinbrook, 1985). Hospitals have yet to resolve such conflicts with clear and consistent policy. Steinbrook et al. (1985) also discuss declining morale and high stress among AIDS health care workers. They note that house officers caring for AIDS patients often become pessimistic, being more negative than positive about drug therapies and hospital treatments. (Steinbrook et al., 1985).

Historically, hospitals have rarely addressed the potential emotional needs of staff who are exposed to death and protracted illness on a daily basis. With AIDS, however, the psychological well-being of medical personnel may finally have to be addressed. Volberding describes a possible solution to staff "burnout" (Iglehart, Read, and Wells, 1987). It involves temporarily replacing exhausted and demoralized staff with practicing physicians who are seeking intense training with AIDS. The latter physicians can then return to their communities with enhanced confidence and ability to treat AIDS, while the hospital physicians they relieved will presumably benefit from the respite.

The testing issue

The CDC claims there is no evidence of HIV transmission from staff to patients (CDC, 1985). Hospitals currently do not routinely require testing of staff for HIV, although physicians often raise the issue (Conte, 1983). The CDC recommends against routine testing of health care workers unless they perform invasive procedures. Also, the CDC recommends against reassigning seropositive health care workers away from direct patient care, unless they have open wounds or treat a patient who has open wounds (*Hospitals,* January 5, 1986). The CDC also recommends that testing be available to staff who request it.

Hospitals seem to be reacting to the CDC recommendations in diverse ways. A University of California at San Francisco task force, setting hospital guidelines for AIDS treatment, states that employees with AIDS must be dealt with individually to determine their risk of transmitting HIV and risk of acquiring an infectious disease from patients (Conte, 1983). The task force also states that hospitals should be allowed to reassign employees with AIDS to positions not involving patient care, for the protection of both workers and patients.

Apparently, relatively few physicians are interested in knowing their HIV status (Link et al., 1988). Physicians lack confidence in the testing procedures, or feel there is no need for the test because they think they are seronegative. In addition, physicians state that, even if they were seropositive, they would not want to know. Finally, physicians see no reason to prevent seropositive physicians from conducting direct patient care (Link et al., 1988). So, while other professions and fields struggle with the issue of testing employees and the transmission of AIDS in all sorts of settings, medical practitioners appear to be taking a laissez faire stance.

While researchers and physicians agree that the risk of contracting AIDS from a patient is quite small (Ponsford, 1987; *American Medical News,* May 16, 1986; CDC, 1985; Frank, 1986; Hendersen et al., 1986; McCray, 1986; McEvoy, Porter, Mortimer, Simmons, and Shanson, 1987), studies on the subject are not in complete agreement. The Surgeon General warns physicians that emergency rooms and operating rooms may be high-risk settings (*Hospitals,* Dec. 5, 1987). As a result, many hospitals are instituting "universal precautions," as recommended by the CDC (1987). These precautions suggest that health care workers treat all patients as potentially seropositive and avoid contact with all patients' body fluids. Precautions also exist around the use and disposal of sharp items such as scalpels, needles, and syringes, the practice of mouth-to-mouth resuscitation, and the use of gloves and masks (CDC, 1985).

Little is known, however, about how closely hospital staff actually follow CDC guidelines. And while hospital public relations officers claim that hospital staff are practicing these universal precautions, hospital workers recently observed by this author over a twenty-month period do not always adhere to CDC guidelines (Lloyd, 1988). For instance, nurses frequently draw blood while not wearing gloves. More observational work should be conducted in order to assess, and account for, variable patterns of adherence to universal precautions among hospital staff.

Educational programs

In response to staff concerns about AIDS, some hospitals have instituted educational programs to control information and relieve staff anxiety (*Hospitals,* January 5, 1986). One article recommends formal education about HIV transmission and infection control guidelines, with optional personal counseling (Link et al., 1988). Wachter (1986) argues that staff training programs must realistically inform staff of the number of AIDS patients at their hospital. Guidelines for minimizing risk should be included in training. Furthermore, Wachter recommends the establishment of a policy regarding "do not resuscitate" orders for AIDS patients. He encourages frank discussions and optional peer and professional counseling to reduce the stress involved in treating AIDS. He also recommends non-AIDS rotations for relieving staff stress.

Again, there are few studies of the impact and usefulness of educational programs. Obviously, hospitals might be interested in assessing the need for and impact of such educational programs before allocating significant resources to them. Such planning is especially relevant since education did not work to control the spread of venereal diseases among World War I soldiers.

Issues for the Future

Historical examples illustrate that, in responding to new epidemics, medicine and hospitals generally implement impromptu, reactive plans using a limited range of resources. Moreover, they show that conventional hospitals alone are not effective. From Wachter's description (1986) of San Francisco General's model for treating AIDS (probably the most sophisticated program in the U.S.), one can see that hospital treatment for AIDS patients is far from perfected. Physicians' descriptions of the issues they confront when treating AIDS reveal that AIDS, like other epidemics throughout U.S.

history, does not neatly fit the hospital model or the medical model for treating serious illness. As in the treatment of previous epidemics, hospital responses to AIDS are shifting from reactive to proactive stances. The initiation of AIDS clinics, units, and hospitals integrated with community resources are some examples. In addition, a few hospitals are changing their organizational goals and functions, as some physicians and other health care workers entertain the idea of shifting from cures to prevention. If historical examples can be used as predictors, these changes bode well for the future.

Hospitals are finding that, with AIDS, they must deal with at least five of the same issues they have confronted for decades: Who will be treated? Who deserves reimbursement for health care? How are chronic diseases best treated? How can a safe work environment be provided for hospital workers? And, what are the potential psychosocial needs of chronic patients and their health care workers?

Concerning the first issue — who will be treated — hospitals, in the aggregate, demonstrate ambivalence. Whereas some hospitals and health care workers welcome AIDS patients, other hospitals and health care workers indirectly and directly discourage their admission. Few hospital administrators treat AIDS patients as a challenge, as opposed to a social problem. The current hospital response is little improvement over hospital responses to cholera, tuberculosis, and venereal diseases.

Second, to meet the financial burden of treating AIDS, some hospitals are working with insurers, communities, and governments. Such hospitals are the exception, however, not the rule. While changes in financing the treatment of this epidemic are slow, economic forecasts show that hospitals soon will have to seriously confront this issue by necessity, if not by choice. While they were confronted with financial problems, yesterday's hospitals didn't have to deal with the complex payment and organizational systems that characterize their modern counterparts.

Third, hospitals remain, with few exceptions, recalcitrant in their treatment practices for chronic patients. While many health care workers despair at the prospects for hospital treatment of AIDS patients, few health care workers simultaneously question conventional, clinical treatments. Historical examples discussed earlier indicate that such questioning must occur before a breakthrough in AIDS treatment will be achieved.

Fourth, according to current research on AIDS transmission, many hospitals provide low-AIDS-risk environments for their workers. This situation, however, has not arisen entirely intentionally; AIDS is fairly hard to transmit with current hospital practices. If hospitals adopt and act on the CDC guidelines, future AIDS transmission should be further reduced. Advances in medical knowledge make AIDS care much safer than cholera, tuberculosis, and venereal disease care were at comparable points in their progress.

Finally, few hospitals include psychosocial treatment specific to AIDS care for their patients and staff. As with previous treatment of infectious disease, hospitals and medicine still do not generally recognize psychosocial treatment as an important adjunct to clinical treatments.

Perhaps history can help with these five issues facing hospitals treating AIDS patients. For example, swift hospital responses to cholera were effective only with a well-coordinated and powerful public health institution backing them. Ambitious, coordinated efforts among hospitals, medical practitioners, the general public, community groups, and public health officials have been most effective in halting the spread of epidemics.

History also counsels caution on the question of quarantining. While voluntary isolation seems to have benefited tubercular patients, involuntary quarantining did not assist in the battles against venereal disease and cholera. In short, there is not clear historical precedent justifying the quarantining of AIDS patients. The creation and funding of hospitals tailored to the needs of AIDS patients, however, may well be effective, especially when bolstered by widespread community support. Thus, hospitals might do well to devise programs for soliciting community involvement.

In the past, hospital health care workers have rarely welcomed patients with epidemic diseases. In fact, many hospitals directly and indirectly discouraged such admissions. Such practices remain today, and are clearly counterproductive. Therefore, hospitals might try to devise programs to recruit health care workers and administrators who want, or at least consider it part of their professional duty, to treat people with AIDS.

Finally, responses to tuberculosis were effective when they were created in alliance with tubercular patients and met patients' psychological needs. While many hospitals have integrated medical and psychological treatments for AIDS, others have not. Health care planners need to consider working more closely with AIDS patients.

References

1. *AIDS Alert.* January, 1987. "Incentives encourage nursing homes to open doors to AIDS patients." 2:6.
2. *AIDS Alert.* October, 1986. "Changes in hospital nursing care, earlier releases could cut costs." 1:177–179.
3. *AIDS Alert.* March, 1986. "AIDS 'Unknowns' have paramedics fearing on-the-job infection risk." 1:61.
4. Ake, J.M. and Lori M. Perlstein. 1987. "AIDS: impact on neuroscience nursing." *Journal of Neuroscience Nursing* 19:300–4.
5. *American Medical News.* "NIH Health workers won't get AIDS from patients." May 16, 1986, 29:12.
6. *American Medical News.* "AIDS patients need more nursing time." March 21, 1986, 29:30.
7. *American Medical News.* "U.S. Must deal with AIDS as public policy." February 7, 1986, 29:22.
8. *American Medical News.* "AIDS risk to health workers minimized." December 6, 1985, 28:2,9.
9. *American Medical News.* "AIDS costs battering hospitals." November 15, 1985, 28:2,27.
10. *American Medical News.* "Citing fears of AIDS transmission, MD stops performing artificial insemination." November 8, 1985, 28:19.
11. *American Medical News.* "AIDS risk troubles MDs, Dr. Volberding reports." October, 18, 1985, 28:3.
12. Andrulis, D.P., Virginia S. Beers, James D. Bentley, and Larry S. Gage. 1987. "The provision and financing of medical care for AIDS patients in U.S. public and private teaching hospitals." *Journal of the American Medical Association* 258:1343–1346.
13. Banks, Taunya Lovell. 1987. "The right to medical treatment." pp. 175–184 in *AIDS and the Law,* edited by Harlon L. Dalton, Scott Burris, and the Yale AIDS Law Project. New Haven and London: Yale University Press.
14. Benfer, David W. "Health care policy issues related to AIDS: lessons learned from the Henry Ford Hospital experience." *Henry Ford Hospital Medical Journal* 35:52–57.
15. Bloom, David E. and Geoffrey Carliner. 1988. "The economic impact of AIDS in the United States." *Science* 239:604–609.
16. Brandt, Allan M. 1987. *No Magic Bullet.* New York, Oxford: Oxford University Press.
17. Centers for Disease Control. 1987. "Recommendations for prevention of HIV transmission in health-care settings." *Morbidity and Mortality Weekly Report* (supplement) 36: 3S–18S.

18. Centers for Disease Control. 1985. "Recommendations for preventing transmission of infection with human t-lymphadenopathy-associated virus in the workplace." *Morbidity and Mortality Weekly Report* 34:681–685,691–694.
19. Conte, J.E., Jr., W. Keith Hadley, Merle Sande, and the University of California, San Francisco, Task Force on the Acquired Immunodeficiency Syndrome. 1983. "Infection-control guidelines for patients with the acquired immunodeficiency syndrome (AIDS)." *New England Journal of Medicine* 309:740–744.
20. DuBos, Rene and Jean DuBos. 1952. The White Plague: *Tuberculosis, Man and Society*. Boston: Little Brown and Company.
21. Frank, Hugh. 1986. "AIDS – the responsibility of health care workers to assume some degree of personal risk." (letter to the editor) *The Western Journal of Medicine*, 144:363–364.
22. Green, Jesse, Madeleine Singer, Neil Wintfeld, Kevin Schulman, and Leigh Passman. 1987. "Projecting the impact of AIDS on hospitals." *Health Affairs* 6:19–31.
23. Groopman, J.E. and A.S. Detsky. 1983. "Epidemic of the acquired immunodeficiency syndrome: a need for economic and social planning." *Annals of Internal Medicine* 99:259–261.
24. Henderson, D.K., Alfred J. Saah, Barbara J. Zak, Richard A. Kaslow, H. Clifford Lane, Thomas Folks, William C. Blackwelder, James Schmitt, Deborah J. LaCamera, Henry Masur, and Anthony Fauci. 1986. "Risk of nomosocial infection with human T-cell lymphotropic virus type III/lymphadenopathy-associated virus in a large cohort of intensively exposed health care workers." *Annals of Internal Medicine* 104:644–647.
25. *Hospitals*. December 5, 1987. "Koop: AIDS poses ethical dilemmas for physicians." 61:61–2.
26. *Hospitals*. January 5, 1986. "AIDS: a time bomb at hospitals' door." 60:54–61,69–70.
27. Green, Jesse et al. 1987. "Projecting the impact of AIDS on hospitals." *Health Affairs* 6:19–31.
28. Iglehart, John K., J. Leighton Read, and James A. Wells. 1987. "The socioeconomic impact of AIDS on health care systems." *Health Affairs* 6:137–147.
29. Kim, J.H. and John R. Perfect. 1988. "To help the sick: an historical and ethical essay concerning the refusal to care for patients with AIDS." *The American Journal of Medicine* 84:135–138.
30. Landesman, S.H., H.M. Ginzburg, and S.H. Weiss. 1985. "Special report: the AIDS epidemic." *New England Journal of Medicine* 312:521–525.
31. Link, R.N., Anat Feinbold, Mitchell H. Charap, Katherine Freeman, and Steven P. Shelov. 1988. "Concerns of medical and pediatric house officers about acquiring AIDS from their patients." *American Journal of Public Health* 78:455–459.
32. Lloyd, R. 1988. "Field notes for NIJ grant." University of California, Santa Barbara.
33. Loewy, E.H. 1986. "AIDS and the physician's fear of contagion." *Chest* 89:325–326.
34. McCray, E. 1986. "The Cooperative Needlestick Surveillance Group: occupational risk of the acquired immunodeficiency syndrome among health care workers." *New England Journal of Medicine* 314:1127–1132.

35. McEvoy, M., Kholoud Porter, Philip Mortimer, Norman Simmons, and David Shanson. 1987. "Prospective study of clinical, laboratory, and ancillary staff with accidental exposures to blood or body fluids from patients infected with HIV." *British Medical Journal* 294:1595–1597.
36. Nary, G. 1987. "The AIDS pandemic: ethical and financial issues [letter]." *Quality Review Bulletin* 13:330–331.
37. *New York Times.* "Attitudes that shape the fight against AIDS: even among doctors, an epidemic of fear." June 2, 1985, p. 3.
38. Ponsford, Gerard. 1987. "AIDS in the OR: a surgeon's view." *Canadian Medical Association Journal* 137:1036–1039.
39. Rosenberg, Charles. 1987. *The Care of Strangers: the Rise of America's Hospital System.* New York: Basic Books.
40. Rosenberg, Charles. 1962. *The Cholera Years.* Chicago and London: University of Chicago Press.
41. Rosner, David. 1982. *A Once Charitable Enterprise.* Cambridge, London, New York: Cambridge University Press.
42. Scitovsky, A.A., Mary Cline, and Philip Lee. 1986. "Medical care costs of patients with AIDS in San Francisco." *Journal of the American Medical Association* 256:3103–3106.
43. Seage, G.R., Stewart Landers, M. Anita Barry, Jerome Groopman, George Lamb, and Arnold Epstein. 1986. "Medical care costs of AIDS in Massachusetts." *Journal of the American Medical Association* 256: 3107–3109.
44. Starr, Paul. 1982. *The Social Transformation of American Medicine.* New York: Basic Books Publishers, Inc.
45. Steinbrook, R., Bernard Lo, Jill Tirpack, James Dilley, and Paul Volberding. 1985. "Ethical dilemmas in caring for patients with the acquired immunodeficiency syndrome." *Annals of Internal Medicine* 103:787–790.
46. Wachter, R. M. 1986. "The impact of the acquired immunodeficiency syndrome on medical residency training." *New England Journal of Medicine* 314:177–180.
47. Wachter, R.M., J.M Luce, J. Turner, P. Volberding, and P.C. Hopewell. 1986. "Intensive care of patients with the acquired immunodeficiency syndrome: outcome and changing patterns of utilization." *American Review of Respiratory Disease* (supplement) 133:A183.
48. *Washington Post National Weekly.* "As AIDS spreads, so does discrimination." December 8, 1986, p.10.

Chapter 4

AIDS-Related Competencies of Primary-Care Physicians

Howard E. Freeman
Charles E. Lewis
Christopher R. Corey

IN THE LESS than a decade since Gottlieb and his associates (1981) identified what they referred to as a "new severe acquired cellular immunodeficiency syndrome," AIDS has emerged as the most troublesome worldwide epidemic of modern times. It annually is taking the lives of thousands of persons, requires a major commitment of economic resources, and has confronted nations throughout the world with social and political issues of major consequence. Although estimates of the number of cases and of the costs of care vary, and are more or less alarming, two separate conferences held in 1986[*] predicted that the number of yearly AIDS deaths in the 1990s will be about 275,000 in the U.S., and the cost of care between $8 and $16 billion.

It is impossible to argue away the consequences of AIDS as a short-term matter, or to ignore the urgency of confronting the effects of providing care for HIV-infected per-

---

[*] The Third International Conference on AIDS and the Cool Font Planning Conference, both held in June, 1986.

sons. The prevailing view is that neither effective therapeutic agents nor efficacious vaccines are likely to be available in the near future. Moreover, the idea that community educational programs will reduce the risks of transmission of the virus is an illusion. For example, a study of sexually active adolescents in San Francisco recently found that although perceptions that condoms reduce sexually transmitted diseases were common, they were not reflected in either intentions to use condoms or in actual use (Kegeles, Adler and Irwin, 1988). Additionally, the social and political issues resulting from the AIDS crisis continue to grow in number and intensity. There is rampant disagreement about whether to require either the testing of the general population or of sub-populations for the HIV virus; there are a multitude of views on where AIDS patients should be provided with treatment and terminal care, and on the extent to which heroic interventions should be attempted to prolong their lives. There are serious questions about whether or not HIV-positive persons should be prevented from engaging in various occupational positions and if they fit the definition of a "minority" with respect to social and work discrimination; and there is the issue of the extent to which others in the community should bear the treatment and health insurance costs that are incurred by HIV-positive people. Moreover, there are serious concerns about how to deal with community response to the "AIDS crisis." In contemporary times at least, no other medical problem approaches AIDS in terms of the speed with which it has achieved community-wide visibility and the extent to which it has aroused fear, anxiety, and hostility among various segments of the population.

In this chapter, we review the results of the first two studies of an ongoing program of research on physicians' responses to the AIDS crisis. Both studies were concerned with the AIDS-related knowledge and behavior of primary-care physicians. The focus on primary-care physicians—general practitioners, internists, and family medicine specialists—was based on the premise that they are in a key position to deal with the direct and indirect effects of the AIDS epidemic.

Primary-care physicians, as part of routine care, have an obligation to identify AIDS-symptomatic patients, and an obvious responsibility to either "work up" or refer them for diagnosis. They have an opportunity to assess the level of risk of their patients, depending on life-style, and advise them if they should or should not be tested for the HIV virus. Furthermore, they can personally encourage preventive practices in their patient population and, when called for, refer for counseling those patients who are at high risk. In addition, primary-care physicians are in a key position to relate to patients who have high levels of anxiety about AIDS because they are personally connected with persons who test positive or they share the generalized emotional reactions of community members to the syndrome. Given the seriousness and persistence of the epidemic, and the continual opportunity of primary-care physicians to interface with the general population, it is clear that the effort to improve health providers' AIDS-related competencies is an important component in any attempt, long- or short-term, to control the transmission of the AIDS virus.

An Overview of the Research

The first study was initiated in 1984, some three years after *The New England Journal of Medicine* article by Gottlieb and his associates was published. It was a "research demonstration" effort to examine the competencies of primary-care physicians practicing in Los Angeles County to deal with the AIDS crisis, and to test the effectiveness of a primary-care physician education program designed to increase their competencies.

Because of the findings of the research demonstration effort, we undertook a statewide survey in 1986 to assess the AIDS-related competencies of California's primary-care physicians. The survey used most of the items from the earlier Los Angeles demonstration effort.

The results of our two studies of primary-care physicians have been reported in journal papers (Lewis, Freeman, Kaplan and Corey, 1986; Lewis, Freeman and Corey, 1987, Lewis and Freeman, 1987). The findings of the two studies are that a significant proportion of primary-care physicians are less than fully competent to diagnose AIDS, to provide counseling to high-risk patients, and to give advice on appropriate responses to the AIDS crisis. Further, we found that a specially designed physician education program had extremely limited impact on the AIDS-related behavior of the physicians who participated in the demonstration.

One purpose of this chapter is to provide a summary of the results of our two studies. A second and, to our minds, more important, purpose is to consider the likelihood of modifying the AIDS-related patient care activities of primary-care physicians, given the correlates of AIDS-related competence that we have identified in the two studies. Finally, we speculate on programmatic efforts that might increase their competencies.

The 1984 Study

In 1984, we received funding from the National Institutes of Health to develop a physician education module that would provide primary-care physicians with current information about AIDS. Based upon informal discussions with physicians in the community, topics for the education program were selected. They included the advisability of taking sexual histories that took into account patients' sexual orientation, the availability of tests for the HIV virus, and the rate of false positives. Arrangements were made to allow participants to receive continuing education credit for taking the "course" we offered.

Information was presented in three different formats:

1. Printed material, consisting of a brochure in the form of a stamp album. Sheets of crack-and-peel stickers illustrated the skin lesions of Kaposi's Sarcoma and provided an algorithm for working up a patient suspected of having AIDS.

2. An audiotape with similar content–an eleven-minute "soap opera" entitled "One Man's Practice." Information on taking sexual histories, the epidemiology of AIDS, the risks of acquiring AIDS, and so on was presented through a dialogue between the characters, who were played by professional actors.

3. A videotape with the same content–a twenty-one-minute "national news broadcast," again professionally done. The actors provided epidemiological information as a "weather map," and did "man on the street" interviews about various facets of AIDS.

A representative sample of 635 primary-care physicians in Los Angeles County, drawn from the American Medical Association data tape which contains the names, addresses, and specialties of all licensed physicians, was surveyed by telephone before the educational program was put in place. The survey included a series of measures of primary-care providers' AIDS-related "competence." The key competence measures assessed were the following: whether or not physicians routinely took sexual histories, and if the histories included information on the sexual orientations; their knowledge of "pre-AIDS" (AIDS-Related Complex); their knowledge of screening tests; the appropriateness of their workups of a hypothetical AIDS patient; their knowledge of risk factors for acquiring AIDS; and their counseling practices with patients about risks of acquiring the syndrome through different types of exposures.

As part of the survey, the physicians were asked if they were interested in receiving educational materials about AIDS and AIDS-related health care. They all replied in the affirmative and random sub-groups received one of the three educational modules described above. Approximately four months later, they were reinterviewed by telephone on the AIDS-related measures included in the first survey, excluding those measures for which there was not a reasonable distribution of responses. (For example, almost all of the physicians at the time of the first interview knew who constituted high-risk groups, so this measure was not repeated.)

The results were most discouraging. A major part of the failure of the program was the fact that only a minority of the physicians who received the materials made use of them. This was the case despite the fact that, after the 635 physicians were sent one of the three sets (on a random basis), all had stated they wanted more information about AIDS. The results on participation are summed up in Table 1.

Table 1.   Participation in AIDS Education Programs

	%	No.
Program participation		
Beginning study group	100.0	635
Post-test interview	80.8	513
Beginning study group who used provided educational materials	43.3	635
Post-test interview group who used educational materials	53.6	513
Proportion participating in programs		
Of physicians receiving reading materials	36.4	184
Of physicians receiving audiotape	50.0	154
Of physicians receiving videotape	46.3	175

We began with 635 physicians, all of whom received materials. But only 513 cooperated and were willing to be interviewed the second time. Consequently, we have information about participation in the education program on only about eighty percent of the original study group of 635 physicians. If we presume that most or all of the 122 physicians who did not cooperate in the post-test interview did not take advantage of the educational materials provided, as shown in Table 1, the maximum proportion who participated is forty-three percent. Of the 513 who were interviewed after the materials were provided, only slightly more than one-half reported reading, listening to, or viewing the materials.

Moreover, as shown in Table 2, on two of four key indicators there are no significant differences between participants and non-participants in the program. In one case (knowledge of screening tests) there is a difference of a few percentage points, and in a second (taking sexual histories) there is about a ten percent gain among program participants compared with non-participants.

Table 2. Test Results after Program

	Total Participants in Programs (n = 275)	Reading Program (n = 117)	Audio Program (n = 77)	Video Program (n = 81)	Post-test Results of Non-participants (n = 238)
Sexual History					
Does not usually take history	18.5†	20.5	19.5	14.8	28.9†
Takes history without sexual orientation	37.5	35.0	36.4	42.0	42.4
Takes history including sexual orientation	44.0	44.5	44.1	43.2	33.6
Knowledge of pre-AIDS complex					
Not heard of pre-AIDS	14.9	12.0	14.3	19.8	21.4
Knew of pre-AIDS, and of three or fewer symptoms	39.6	37.6	45.5	37.0	38.7
Knew of pre-AIDS and three or more symptoms	45.5	50.4	40.3	43.2	39.9
Knowledge of screening tests					
Knew no test	15.3†	16.2	13.0	16.0	24.4†
Knew T-cell or HTLV-III test	30.5	29.1	31.2	32.1	25.6
Knew T-cell or HTLV-III test and concerned about false positives	54.2	54.7	55.8	51.9	50.0
Diagnostic work-up of a hypothetical case					
Did not seek appropriate information and/or AIDS not considered in differential diagnosis	21.1	20.5	29.9	13.6	24.8
Obtained sexual history and AIDS considered in diagnosis	58.5	60.7	50.6	63.0	54.2
Obtained sexual history, checked for organomegaly, and AIDS in diagnosis	20.4	18.8	19.5	23.5	21.0

* Pre-post test difference. $p < 0.01$.
† Participants vs. non-participants. $p < 0.05$.

It should be noted that there was, however, considerable secular change between the two time periods, a consequence of the attention paid to AIDS during that period by both the media and professional publications. For example, the number who both knew of a test for the virus and were properly concerned with false positives rose from 19.8 to 52.2 percent.

Of particular note, however, is that when regression analyses were undertaken, the personal and professional characteristics — *not* program participation — of the physicians explained virtually all of the variation in competence. The physician characteristics that were included in the analysis are shown in Table 3. The analysis was undertaken two ways. First, with responses to the dependent variables, i.e., the competence measures, left in three categories as shown in Table 2 and then collapsed into two categories. In collapsed form, the last category shown in Table 2 was compared to pooled responses in the first two. That is, for example, "competence" in terms of sexual history-taking after collapsing refers to taking a sexual history that includes sexual orientation.

Table 3. Regression and Logit Values for Competence Indicators (Post-test)*

	Sexual History-taking R^2 0.12 D Logit 0.23 B / P	Knowledge of Pre-Aids Complex R^2 0.20 D Logit 0.31 B / P	Knowledge of Screening Tests R^2 0.08 D Logit 0.18 B / P	Diagnostic Work-up of a Hypothetical Case R^2 0.06 D Logit 0.20 B / P
Internist (dummy)	0.10 / 0.29	0.36† / 0.93†	0.29† / 1.13†	0.22† / 1.23
Family practice (dummy)	0.19‡ / 0.46	0.08 / 0.23	0.03 / 0.37	0.10 / 0.57
Years in practice	-0.08† / -0.25†	-0.02 / -0.03	-0.01 / 0.05	0.09† / 0.15
Medical school attended	0.03 / 0.02	-0.06 / 0.09	-0.03 / 0.00	0.04 / -0.20
Number of MDs in practice	0.02 / -0.01	0.15† / 0.32†	0.00 / -0.03	0.05 / 0.08
Worked up or referred patients for AIDS	0.04 / 0.04	0.11 / 0.19	0.13 / 0.29	0.01 / 0.22
Have patients concerned about AIDS	0.09‡ / 0.32‡	0.16† / 0.35†	0.08 / 0.18	0.04 / 0.26
Have advised patients on AIDS prevention	0.22† / 0.53†	0.12 / 0.05	0.00 / 0.04	0.03 / -0.12
Have attended lectures on AIDS	0.06‡ / 0.17‡	0.07† / 0.17‡	0.05‡ / 0.17¶	0.03 / -0.11
Believe average MD uncomfortable discussing sexual matters with homosexuals	0.00 / -0.08‡	-0.24‡ / -0.07‡	-0.18 / -0.04	-0.16 / 0.06
Discomfort compared with other doctors at having homosexual patients in practice	0.07 / 0.31*	0.00 / 0.11	-0.03 / -0.12	-0.06 / -0.34‡

* B = unstandardized regression coefficient; p = unstandardized profit coefficient.
† P < 0.01.
‡ P < 0.05.
¶ P < 0.06.

The findings do not differ markedly when least square analyses are undertaken, using the three-way distribution on the four measures of competence or logit regressions with these measures dichotomized as described. Taken together, the ten independent variables explain between six and twenty percent of the variance when estimated from the least square analysis. All of the logit regressions, the "D" values in Table 3, likewise are statistically significant (for a discussion of Somner's D see Harrell, 1983).

The results confirm the cross-tabular analyses that also were undertaken. Specialty and years of practice were significant predictors of most of the measures of knowledge and AIDS-related practices. Internists are the most likely of the three primary-care provider groups to score higher on the measures. The longer the physician has been in practice, the less likely he or she is to be high in competence.

Also, physicians who reported they had worked up a possible AIDS patient, or had given a patient advice on preventive practices, or had patients concerned with AIDS, were more likely to score higher on the measures than those who had not. Finally, questions that tap homophobia are related to several of the outcome measures.

Given the findings, we decided to undertake another study, this time simply a cross-sectional survey in order to continue to monitor physicians' knowledge and practice in relation to AIDS, and to try to replicate the findings on the relations between physician characteristics and knowledge and practice. The results of the "evaluation" strongly suggested the futility of the type of educational effort that we undertook. The results of our evaluation simply produced additional evidence about the low efficacy of physician education programs (see, for example, Egdahl and German, 1977).

The 1986 Survey

In 1986, we undertook a second study with state funds administered by the University of California. Using virtually the same interview schedule as the first of the 1984 surveys, we surveyed—again by telephone—a random sample of 1000 primary-care physicians practicing in the State of California. As before, the sample was drawn from the AMA tape containing information about physicians in the state. The 1986 survey was conducted statewide in order to extend generalization potential of the earlier study with respect to physician characteristics predictive of AIDS-related competence. Moreover, since Los Angeles physicians were a major sub-sample in the 1986 survey, it was possible to examine changes over time in competence for practitioners residing in Los Angeles County. The period between the two studies was one in which AIDS was a continual preoccupation of the mass media and the subject of numerous articles in various medical journals. Thus, one would expect a pronounced secular trend in knowledge and practice behavior.

The 1986 data clearly indicate secular trends in the direction of increased competence to deal with AIDS-related health problems, at least in terms of the majority of the six measures of AIDS-related competence included in the survey. In Table 4, we show the "competence levels" in 1986 and, for physicians practicing in Los Angeles County, in 1984 and 1986 on each of six measures. We regard the proportions reported in the third category on each of the measures to be physicians "high" in competence. For example, if a primary-care physician takes sexual histories from his or her patients, persons of high risk can be identified for diagnostic workups, preventive advice and so on.

Physicians in Los Angeles County, and California in general, were considerably more likely in 1986 to take a sexual history that includes sexual orientation than were Los Angeles practitioners in 1984. Similarly, they were more likely to know about "pre-AIDS" and its symptoms, and to correctly identify low-risk groups. There was no change, however, in their knowledge about the risks of false positives connected with HIV testing, although clearly the proportion that knew about an HIV test rose markedly in the two years between the surveys. They were also more likely in 1986 than 1984 to correctly advise their patients about the low risk of exposure to AIDS when presented with vignettes describing several low-risk interpersonal contact situations.

While the overall findings for California, and time comparisons for physicians in Los Angeles County, reveal increased competence in 1986 compared to 1984, there remained a significant proportion of physicians even in 1986 whose AIDS-related competence was questionable. Of course, any definition of competence is arbitrary. Yet, even some five years after the syndrome had been identified, and despite significant attention to AIDS in both the medical and popular literature, there is serious reason to be concerned with the practice behavior and knowledge of primary-care physicians on AIDS-related matters. For California as a whole, the key findings are as follows:

1. Only thirty-five percent of the physicians report routinely taking sexual histories that include sexual orientation.

2. Less than one-half were aware both of the AIDS-related complex (ARC) and of four or five of its key symptoms.

3. Only sixteen percent knew both of appropriate tests for AIDS and of the critical need to be concerned with the specificity of these tests.

4. Less than twenty percent correctly worked up a hypothetical case in which AIDS was a reasonable differential diagnosis.

5. Only slightly more than one-half of the physicians correctly identified more than four risk factors generally held to involve low risks of infection.

Table 4. Primary Care Physicians' AIDS-Related Behavior and Knowledge

		Los Angeles	
Measures	State % 1986	1986	1984
Sexual History Taking			
No sexual history usually taken	16.9	15.8	27.9
Sexual history taken but does not include sexual orientation	48.1	40.9	45.7
Sexual history taken that includes sexual orientation	35.0	43.4	26.5
Knowledge of Pre-AIDS Complex			
Not heard of Pre-AIDS Complex	28.0	28.0	43.5
Knew about pre-AIDS but could cite three or less symptoms	27.3	26.9	24.1
Knew about Pre-AIDS and cited four or five symptoms	44.7	45.2	32.4
Knowledge of Screening Tests			
Knew no tests	18.2	14.0	72.0
Knew T-Cell or HTLV-III tests	65.4	65.9	8.2
Knew T-Cell or HTLV-III tests and concerned with false positives	16.4	20.1	19.8
Diagnostic Work-up of Hypothetical Case			
Did not seek appropriate information and/or AIDS not differential diagnosis	44.4	44.8	50.7
Obtained sexual history or appropriate physical examination and AIDS a diagnosis	38.0	38.4	32.9
Obtained both sexual history and physical examination and AIDS a diagnosis	17.6	16.8	16.4
Correctly identify Low-Risk Exposure Groups			
Identified none or one low-risk factors	18.1	22.2	32.1
Identified two low-risk factors	10.7	12.5	25.0
Identified three low-risk factors	18.5	19.7	20.8
Identified four to eight low-risk factors	52.8	45.5	21.6
Correctly Advise Patients of Low-Risk of Exposure to AIDS			
Correct in no cases	12.7	13.3	39.4
Correct in one to two cases	53.1	55.6	28.5
Correct in three cases or four cases	34.1	32.1	32.1
100% equals	1000	350	635

At best, these percentages provide an estimate of the maximum AIDS-related competence of the physicians interviewed. It is highly unlikely, for example, that physicians who take sexual histories that include sexual orientation would report otherwise, but the reverse may not be so. Indeed, a 1988 survey of a representative sample of persons in Los Angeles County—1138 adults—conducted by the Institute for Social Science Research of UCLA, asked the 990 who had visited a physician within the past three years whether, on any occasion, they were asked about past sexual contacts. As shown in Table XX, only fourteen percent had had a sexual history taken that included sexual orientation. Interestingly, the percent who had a sexual history taken is lower for men than for women, and also lower for persons with incomes over $30,000. If anything, then, as low as it is, the reports we obtained from physicians represent a maximum estimate of the proportion of people about whose sexual histories (a key indicator of life-style in relation to AIDS) physicians are aware.

Table 4a. Percent of Los Angeles County Adults Asked About Sexual Contacts (with M.D. visits in three years.)

Total Sample	14.4%
Males	11.3
Females	17.0
Income under $30,000	19.6
Income $30,000 and over	11.0

Of particular note, as in the 1984 survey, there were systematic relationships between the personal and professional characteristics of physicians and their AIDS-related competence. As shown in Table 5, at the bivariate level most of the predictor variables are associated with the competence measures. In this table, the competence measures were dichotomized so that the percentages reflect the percent in the last category; i.e., the high competence category on each of the measures as listed in Table 4. For example, on the sexual history measure, taking a history that includes sexual orientation is associated with being an internist, being in practice fewer years, having four or more associates in the practice, practicing in Los Angeles, having worked up patients with AIDS, having patients concerned about AIDS, having attended lectures on AIDS, and not reporting being uncomfortable with having homosexuals in the practice.

Table 5. AIDS Competence Measures and Physician Characteristics

Physical Characteristics	Sexual History Taking	Knowledge of Pre-Aids	Knowledge of Screening Test	Diagnostic Work-up	Identification Risk Groups	Advise Patients Correctly	100%
Total	35.0	44.7	16.4	17.6	52.8	34.1	1000
Specialty							
General Practice	26.5	31.2	12.3	10.0	41.2	27.6	178
Family Medicine	30.8	39.5	16.3	16.6	55.4	36.5	470
Internal Medicine	43.6	56.7	18.5	22.1	54.8	34.3	352
No. Years in Practice							
5 or Less	43.5	53.1	20.1	22.1	57.8	47.8	222
6-15	36.3	53.0	17.7	22.0	55.5	37.3	310
16-30	32.8	38.5	15.0	14.4	54.3	27.6	309
31 and over	25.6	30.3	12.1	9.8	38.0	22.7	159
Medical School Attended							
Excellent	37.4	48.8	15.8	14.3	64.1	32.9	207
Superior	32.2	40.6	19.1	19.6	52.2	37.6	389
Good or Average	36.2	52.0	13.6	19.4	48.8	40.0	233
LDC - Foreign	36.3	38.7	16.9	12.6	45.3	19.4	127
No. of MDs in Practice							
One	27.5	36.7	14.0	17.2	49.5	27.1	528
Two-Three	39.1	53.1	20.0	16.0	56.4	43.1	214
Four or More	46.4	53.6	18.4	19.7	56.2	40.9	258
Region							
Los Angeles	43.4	45.2	20.1	16.8	45.5	31.2	279
San Francisco	34.0	48.2	12.2	17.8	59.9	34.5	197
Other SMSAs	27.5	42.2	16.1	19.4	53.1	37.0	211
Non-SMSAs	29.7	40.3	16.3	14.1	58.5	35.5	313
Worked up Patients w/AIDS							
No Cases	30.9	38.2	14.3	15.8	51.1	30.0	682
One or More Cases	42.5	56.4	19.6	20.4	56.0	41.4	315
Have Patients Concerned about AIDS							
None or only low-risk	26.3	36.5	15.2	17.1	49.2	29.3	478
Patients at risk	35.2	43.7	17.5	16.2	53.1	37.3	315
Patients at visit with symptoms	50.2	60.5	17.2	20.4	58.5	38.4	207
Patients Have Attended Lectures on AIDS							
0	22.1	29.4	15.9	12.9	51.7	28.4	271
1	33.4	41.5	20.1	17.1	51.1	40.4	195
2	36.9	46.6	15.6	16.5	52.1	37.9	222
3 or More	43.1	55.3	15.6	21.8	54.7	32.2	312
Discomfort Compared with Colleagues of having Homosexuals in Practice							
Little	37.3	47.3	18.1	18.8	54.4	37.8	819
Moderate	23.5	34.6	11.4	11.2	43.0	20.2	126
A Good Deal	21.0	24.5	8.5	11.7	51.3	12.8	32

Multiple regression analyses were undertaken between the three-way classifications of the six competency measures and personal and professional characteristics of physicians. A significant regression coefficient is obtained on each of the measures, although because of the intercorrelations between independent variables, many of the measures statistically significant at the zero-order level are not significant in the regressions. The same findings hold when logit analyses were undertaken with the dependent variables dichotomized so that only fully appropriate reports of behavior and knowledge are classified as "competent."

In addition, a "total competence score" was obtained by summing up the number of measures on which a physician scored in the "high competence" category. The distribution on this "index" is skewed in the incompetence direction. Almost eleven percent of the study group failed to score in the competence category on any of the six individual measures; in contrast only two percent scored in the competence category on five or six of the measures. A logit analysis was undertaken in which all of the physician characteristics discussed earlier were included (with the two highest competent categories collapsed). The results are shown in Table 6.

AIDS-Related Competencies of Primary-Care Physicians

Table 6. Logit Analysis of Predictors of "Overall Competence"

Physician Characteristics	Beta	P<*
Have Concerned Patients	.253	.0007
No. of Lectures Attended	.257	.0000
No. of Physicians in Practice	.258	.0002
Discomfort Having Gay Patients	.071	.0493
Average Physician's Discomfort	.184	.0007
Urban/Rural Location	.144	.1317
Specialty	.346	.0000
School	.108	.0017
Years in Practice	.494	.0000

Somner's D = .372

* one-tailed test

All the measures, except for the rural-urban measure, are related to the overall competence measure. What is not revealed by the findings presented in this table are the time-ordered, i.e., "causal," linkages between the independent variables. Since we did not begin with an explicit causal model, it is only possible to suggest how these variables are so related to each other.

A version of the linkages between the independent variables is shown in Figure 1, the result of an *ex post facto* path analysis. The path analysis should be viewed as highly tentative (and consequently the regression coefficients are not shown); it suffers from the simplification of excluding non-recursive relationships, as well as the use of a least square solution with variables that are mostly ordinal and often skewed.

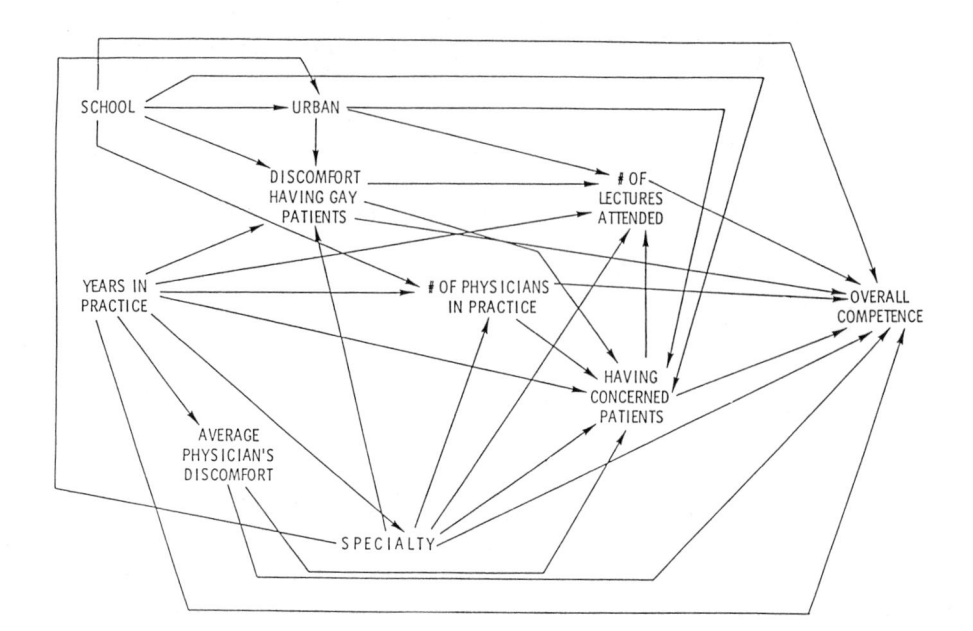

Figure 1. Hypothesized Determinants of AIDS-Related Competence

Nevertheless, our results do allow us to offer the following set of hypotheses:

1. Physicians may learn about AIDS by attending lectures and seminars about AIDS, or because their practices include patients concerned about AIDS. These are the most proximal causes; lecture and seminar attendance, however, is hypothesized to be a possible consequence, but not a cause, of having patients who are concerned about AIDS.

2. Physicians' attitudes towards homosexuals are presumed to affect competence because they are a determinant of the composition of their practices (or their sensitivity to having Gay patients) and also of their likelihood of attending lectures and seminars.

3. Physicians' practice arrangements, in terms of number of colleagues, are hypothesized to be related to attending lectures and seminars and to contact with AIDS-concerned patients. The former relationship is hypothesized because group practices may provide more time for participating in professional education efforts; the latter because large practices (including HMOs) usually have more heterogeneous patient populations, and thus an increased chance of contact with either high risk or concerned patients.

4. Specialty training is viewed as four things: a determinant of attending lectures and seminars (because of the increased emphasis on ac-

quiring knowledge which occurs during socialization as a specialist); as a predictor of contact with AIDS-concerned patients (because of referrals to physicians and the increased likelihood they would work up the "unusual cases," rather than referring them out of their practices); as a correlate of number of physicians in their practices (because of the increased likelihood of general practitioners to opt for solo practice); and as associated with homophobic attitudes (because of their *presumed* increased educational and "cosmopolitan" experiences).

5. Whether or not a physician's practice is located in an urban area is believed to affect a physician's attitudes toward Gays, as does the composition of their patient population, their access to continuing education, and the number of physicians in the practice. It also possibly directly affects AIDS-related competence (if the practice is in an urban center there are more opportunities for peer contact and information exchange). Specialty choice and medical school can be seen as precursors to practice location, as they temporally precede this choice. Further, we assume that those who attended more prestigious medical schools were more likely to seek careers in urban areas, where opportunities congruent with their training are available. Years of practice was seen as affecting location of practice, by virtue of the changes in opportunities in urban areas over the years.[1]

6. The prestige (or quality) of the medical school attended, and years of practice are hypothesized to be related to all of the independent predictors discussed. These two measures are viewed as exogenous variables since, in their influence on the other predictors (and of course directly on competence), they are distal to the other measures but inseparable from each other. Given the ad hoc nature of the path model, we have ignored possible non-recursive relationships between independent variables.

While not all of the suggested relationships discussed above may hold up upon replication — and the direction of the relationships and ordering of the variables may need some revision — the general thesis appears reasonable: competence in AIDS-related practices and knowledge are directly and indirectly rooted in physicians' personal and professional backgrounds, including quite distal and immutable characteristics such as type of medical school attended, specialty choice, and length of time in practice.

Conclusions

Given the findings of our two studies, and to the extent that the suggested relationships between the variables included in the analyses pertain, there is reason to be pessimistic about primary-care physicians having the competencies to realize the key role they might play in the control and prevention of AIDS. Certainly there is little reason to believe that their ordinary professional experiences during their day-to-day work lives can provide them with the competencies necessary to deal with AIDS-related medical care matters. Likewise, it is not possible to expect conventional continuing education efforts to remedy gaps in physicians' "competence" to deal with AIDS and its medical and social ramifications. As we have learned, it is clearly simplistic to believe that merely providing attractively packaged information via audio and video tapes will result in marked increases in medical knowledge and practices. Rather, if primary-care physicians are to maximize their opportunities to deal with AIDS as a medical and sociopolitical problem, innovative means are required to provide them with new information as it emerges from laboratory and clinical research, and particularly to modify their AIDS-related patient care behavior.

Of course, when our findings from the 1984 and 1986 studies are compared, secular changes in knowledge do occur, and to some extent there is changed practice behavior as well. But as there was a significant proportion of physicians not taking appropriate sexual histories in 1986 (and many still are not doing so), it is doubtful that the large majority of physicians, during patient visits, are currently actively advocating the regular use of condoms for those at moderate or high risk of acquiring AIDS. It is also doubtful that they are providing contemporary information about the transmission of AIDS in work places and social settings. To put it bluntly, the secular changes in knowledge that are occurring among primary-care physicians probably are not much different from those taking place among regular readers of *Time* or *Newsweek*. And the pace at which physicians' practice behavior is changing is probably again no greater than the speed at which sexual practice and life-style changes are occurring among the general population.

Our findings may be useful in developing new approaches to increasing the AIDS-related competencies of primary-care physicians. For example, physicians who have been in practice the longest are *least* likely to score high in competence. These physicians also seem to have the least contact with patients concerned about AIDS and are less likely to have worked up AIDS cases. To the extent that their lack of AIDS-related practice experience is related to the characteristics of the patients they routinely treat, it may be possible to organize clinical experiences for them that would reorient their outlooks.

For example, given the critical nature of the epidemic, despite the costs, the idea of bringing clinical training to solo and group practitioners might be considered. It might involve having an infectious disease specialist experienced in the diagnosis and treatment of AIDS, along with one or more actual patients, actually arrange to visit providers' offices and observe "workups" undertaken there. Indeed, well-informed ARC and AIDS patients might be willing to volunteer time to make visits on request, giving physicians an opportunity to discuss AIDS-related issues with them. Practitioners may be able to glean considerable useful information from this, in the same way they are believed to have learned from the now-rarely-seen medical detail man.

Another finding is that American general practitioners and physicians trained in medical schools in lesser-developed countries are least likely to score high in competence. Such physicians generally see high numbers of patients per work day and charge lower fees. Certainly this is the case for those whose patients are on Medicaid or otherwise limited in ability to pay. For example, for such physicians to take even the five to ten minutes per patient required to obtain a sexual history would mean income loss, a prospect which may be a disincentive to history-taking. It might be useful to evaluate whether or not reimbursement for AIDS-related activities would be an incentive for physicians, particularly those treating low-income populations, to increase their AIDS-related competencies and to undertake appropriate practice behavior.

What is clear is that primary-care physicians, although in a key position to contribute to the control and prevention of AIDS and to reduce the uncertainty, anxiety, and questionable political reactions of the general population, are in many cases not doing so, and do not have the competencies to do so. Primary-care physicians represent a resource that must be used to control and prevent AIDS, and to manage the direct and indirect psychological, social, and political consequences of the epidemic. The crisis simply is too serious not to fully and appropriately utilize the large cadre of primary-care physicians in the battle against AIDS.

References

1. Gottlieb, M.S., J.D. Weisman, P.T. Fan, H.S. Schanker, R.A. Wolf, A. Saxon. 1981. "Pneumocystis Carinii Pneumonia and Mucosal Candidiasis in Previously Healthy Homosexual Men: Evidence for a New Severe Acquired Cellular Immunodeficiency Syndrome." *New England Journal of Medicine* 305:1, 425–31.
2. Harrell, F.E., Jr. 1983. "The Logist Procedure." *SAS Applications Guide,* Cary, North Carolina, SAS Institute, Inc.
3. Kegeles, S.M., N.E. Adler, C.E. Irwin. 1988. "Sexually Active Adolescents and Condoms: Changes Over One Year in Knowledge, Attitudes and Use." *American Journal of Public Health* 78:4, 460–461.
4. Lewis, C.E., H.E. Freeman, S.H. Kaplan, C.R. Corey. 1986. "The Impact of a Program to Enhance the AIDS-Related Competencies of Primary care Physicians." *Journal of General Internal Medicine* 1:287–294.
5. Lewis, C.E., H.E. Freeman, C.R. Corey. 1987. "AIDS-Related Competence of California's Primary care Physicians." *American Journal of Public Health* 77:7, 795–799.
6. Lewis, C.E., H.E. Freeman. 1987. "The Sexual History-Taking and Counseling Practices of Primary care Physicians." *The Western Journal of Medicine* Aug:147, 165–167.

Chapter 5

AIDS and the Catholic Church

Alice Horrigan

"WE'RE IN A SITUATION of life and death," said Father Arturo Gomez, pastor of Our Lady Queen of Angels Church in East Los Angeles. "Are we going to believe God can help us or not?" The priest was speaking, in Spanish, to hundreds of Latino parishioners gathered for Sunday Mass during Memorial Day weekend, 1988. The subject of his homily: SIDA, or – as the fatal disease is known in English – AIDS.

Latino families represent seven percent of the U.S. population, yet they suffer with fourteen percent of all AIDS cases.[1] Father Gomez explained the gravity of the epidemic to the Latino men, women, and children crowding the pews and aisles, and called for compassion for those afflicted with AIDS. He asked for help in the battle against ignorance and hysteria. "For the love of God," he urged, parents must guide their children in sexuality. "We need more people in this struggle."

Many AIDS activists suggest that Latinos lag five years behind the rest of the population in their awareness of the disease. When he finished, Father Gomez handed the microphone to a youthful Latino man suffering from AIDS. Armando Rios described to

---

[1] See Hopkins (1987).

the hundreds of Spanish-speaking worshipers the symptoms of his AIDS-related Kaposi's Sarcoma. He explained that the disease is not a punishment from God, as many believe.[2] He has lived with AIDS this long (two and a half years since diagnosis), he said, because "God is helping me — he's helping me every day." When Rios finished, the room sounded with applause and many people were teary-eyed. On the church steps, AIDS education activists from various organizations distributed leaflets in Spanish. "This is a special day," beamed one pamphleteer. "The Church has never done this before."

Indeed, for the first time several nonsectarian institutions had joined in a highly public, cooperative effort with the Roman Catholic Church to combat the AIDS epidemic in the Los Angeles Latino community. From 6:00 a.m. to 8:00 p.m. that Sunday, an hourly Spanish mass was dedicated to AIDS; its message — and the educational talks in the courtyard between services — reached an estimated 9,000 people. The event was a milestone in Latino AIDS education in Los Angeles, a goal only recently imagined possible. Says Zoila Escobar, bilingual health educator and one of the organizers of the day, "If six months ago you had tried to convince people this would happen they would have said, 'Yeah, yeah, you've got to be kidding!'"

Escobar's comment illustrates how the AIDS crisis may be rapidly changing the face of society: physically, economically, institutionally, sexually, and spiritually. This chapter explores — and intends to help direct — a key element of that change: the joint efforts between the Catholic Church and non-sectarian institutions in AIDS programs directed toward Latinos.[3]

We know that in the United States AIDS impacts disproportionately upon minorities. Blacks and Latinos are mourning larger numbers of their Gay community members, heterosexuals, and infants. Special efforts are needed to reach these populations. Among Latinos, especially in the realm of the family, perhaps the most powerful institution is the Roman Catholic Church. As the crowded mass at Our Lady Queen of Angels Church (the largest Latino parish in the Los Angeles Archdiocese) demonstrated, the Church can be a powerful resource, especially for Latinos, in society's mobilization against AIDS.[4]

The first part of this chapter discusses the logistical and ideological power of the Catholic Church to impact the beliefs and behaviors of its followers. The second part focuses on the response of the Los Angeles Archdiocese — the largest in the country —

---

[2] In an April 1987 Gallup Survey, forty-three percent of Latinos agreed with the statement, "Most people with AIDS have only themselves to blame." Latinos were also more likely than others to consider AIDS a "moral punishment." (Gallup)

[3] The mainstream appellation for people of Spanish, Portugese, or Latin American background is "Hispanic." This term, however, lionizes the Spanish heritage while disregarding the *indigenous* roots of those with Latin American lineage. A substitute word gaining popluarity is "Latino." This recognizes the common denominator of Romance languages while also evoking the autonomous character of Latin America. This paper thus employs the term "Latino," except of course when people quoted have used the word "Hispanic."

[4] An estimated eighty-five percent of Latinos in the United States are Catholic. Significant numbers of Latinos also also belong to protestant sects, such as the Baptists, Jehovah's Witnesses, the Church of Jesus Christ of Latter-Day Saints (Mormons), and the Pentecostal (Charismatic Movement) churches. A SIECUS report notes additional Latino affiliation with "alternate" religions such as "Espiritismo" and "Santerismo" (SIECUS): Additional research would be valuable on the role of these churches, especially the popular and often very progressive Protestant ones, in the battle against AIDS.

to the AIDS crisis. It details the ministerial and educational efforts of the Archdiocese, and places them in their national context.

Part three turns to the central questions: how strong are—and should be—the linkages between Church and nonsectarian efforts? By examining the linkages between the Los Angeles Archdiocese and the region's nonsectarian institutions, this section explores how the Church's ideological and spiritual positions can be reconciled with those of other groups.

Finally, what are the implications of AIDS for the Church itself? Will intensification of the crisis carry the Church over the threshold of far-reaching theological change? This part looks at the issues confronting Catholicism in the AIDS crisis, and speculates on their theological and political implications.

The conclusion presents recomendations directed toward both the Church and nonsectarian organizations for more effectively combatting the AIDS epidemic in Latino communities.

THE POTENTIAL OF THE CATHOLIC CHURCH

Experts widely accept that the "second wave" of the AIDS epidemic will seriously threaten the minority communities and compound their present reality: AIDS already has a disproportionate impact on minority populations in the United States. While the disease itself is no less devastating for the Anglo population, it thickens the layers of additional problems already faced by Blacks and Latinos; in minority communities, AIDS is affecting proportionately more heterosexuals and children[5] (see Appendix A).

The Latino population is one context in which we must recognize the importance of the Catholic Church. "Organized religion wields tremendous influence and power in society," notes the self-care manual prepared by the Spiritual Advisory Committee of AIDS Project Los Angeles (APLA). "It can marshal enormous resources of personnel (paid and volunteer), money, and institutions to meet social needs, often more quickly and more efficiently than government agencies and programs can" (SAC).

Yet articles on AIDS often refer only briefly to the influence of the Catholic Church in Latino communities. A report on Latino culture and sex education by the Sex Information and Education Council of the U.S. (SIECUS), for instance, dedicates a mere paragraph to religion. "The practice of religion is deeply imbedded in the Latino cul-

---

[5] Disease generally affects lower classes the most. "It is evident that low socioeconomic status is most strikingly associated with high rates of infectious and parasitic diseases...," write Leonard Syme and Lisa Berkman in the *American Journal of Epidemiology* (see Syme, 1978). Studies have shown that populations in lower-class groups and with low educational levels have excess mortality rates and higher morbidity rates (including susceptibility to mental illness and hypertension). Most studies confirm that social class, more than race or any other factor, is responsible for the higher mortality rates and susceptibility to disease. Studies attempting to identify the principal reason for this class gap have focused on three concerns: lower classes have little access to health care, live in "more toxic, hazardous and non-hygienic environments," and have higher stress and less healthy "coping" styles, which affect general susceptibility to disease.

ture," it notes. "Approximately 85 percent of all Latinos are Catholic"; yet, the report suggests, Catholic action around AIDS has been minimal.

That the religious cornerstone of diverse Latino cultures is deserving of more attention is clear when one considers the extent to which the Catholic Church is linked with these populations. Latinos vary in their cultural customs and values, race, social class, and educational levels, but they have one commonality: most of them are associated with the Roman Catholic Church, either directly or through extended family networks.

Catholics listen to weekly sermons, attend catechism, receive marriage counseling, visit confessionals, attend parochial schools, and participate in youth groups, retreats, and many Church organizations. An army of Catholic priests, nuns, brothers, and laity are a daily influence on Latino lives, providing spiritual guidance and many practical services. Since the AIDS crisis requires discussion about sexuality, and the Church maintains sexuality in the realm of the sacred, it could be argued that the Church is in the best position to provide AIDS education to Latino faithful.

In addition to its human resource infrastructure, the Catholic Church has tremendous logistical advantage over many other organizations: it has substantial budgets and physical facilities, strong national and international communications networks, established programs and community organizations designed to target specific groups, and hundreds of elementary and high schools. The Church's relatively independent parish system, meanwhile, promotes sensitivity to the unique conditions and needs of individual communities. Finally, the Church holds something that both government and nonsectarian institutions lack—spiritual authority. This authority is exercised through its multitude of communications vehicles, such as Sunday homilies, radio and television programs, and publications.

For example, the Catholic Church directs two national television networks: the Catholic Telecommunications Network of America and the Eternal Word Television Network (the latter's programs are transmitted directly through cable companies).[6] Several religious orders run their own communications companies, while individual clergy, nuns, brothers, and lay people produce talk shows for radio and television. Print media, such as the *National Catholic Reporter,* the *Register,* and Catholic magazines are also significant outlets of information.

Individual dioceses, meanwhile, have their own information systems. The Telecommunications Department of the Los Angeles Archdiocese runs an instructional television station with three channels connected to eighty-five of its 228 elementary schools. It also publishes a weekly newspaper and maintains a Public Affairs office that acts as a liaison with other, including non-Catholic, media. A massive study of the communications needs of the Latino population is being launched by the Archdiocese through its Telecommunications Department. If completed, such a study could be an indispensable tool for coordinating AIDS outreach efforts.

Even without much hard data, we can safely conclude that the potential for the Church to reach Latinos with AIDS education is immense. But to what degree does the Church itself recognize this potential and its obligations in the crisis?

---

[6] The Eternal Word Television Network, according to Sister Jeanne Harris of the Los Angeles Archdiocese Telecommunications Department, is very conservative—"almost fundamentalist." The network recently rejected an AIDS education program produced by an independent group of Catholic laity at Santa Fe Communications in Burbank. This does not, however, necessarily eliminate the network's potential for providing basic AIDS education; nor does it reflect on the Church as a whole.

MOBILIZATION OF THE LOS ANGELES ARCHDIOCESE

To understand the context within which the Los Angeles Archdiocese (LAA)[7] is mobilizing against AIDS, it is useful to understand how the Catholic hierarchy conceptualizes its "calling" in the crisis. The word "compassion" perhaps best summarizes the Catholic approach to people whose lives are affected by AIDS. According to the bishops of the California Catholic Conference (CCC), in their May 1987 pastoral letter entitled *A Call to Compassion,* people with AIDS are "sisters and brothers of Jesus, and bear a special resemblance to Him because of their suffering."

The California Catholic Conference

The CCC pastoral letter is an important document that guides priests, nuns, brothers, and lay people in their struggle with AIDS in California's diverse parishes. Christians are responsible, the bishops emphasize, not only for informing themselves about the disease and working towards its prevention, but for caring for those stricken. The bishops recommend reading the Surgeon General's Report on AIDS, but call for a "spiritual interpretation" of the document. "Like all technical studies which touch on such intimate and sacred areas as human sexuality," say the bishops, "the report needs to be studied in a moral context" (CCC:2).

The media has well publicized this "moral context," which recommends sexual abstinence before marriage, monogamous fidelity within marriage, and avoidance of illicit drugs. "The recovery of the virtue of chastity," suggest the bishops, "may be one of the most urgent needs of contemporary society"(CCC:2).

The bishops urge the following actions. Church workers and members should offer prayer, companionship, and assistance to people with AIDS, and reach out to the homosexual community ("We suggest special training to make caregivers more sensitive to the needs of this group" (CCC:3)). Catholic hospitals and community-based organizations should exhibit leadership in health care of AIDS patients, health providers and pastoral ministers should engage in collaborative research and reflection on how to counsel women about sexual activity and prenatal and obstetric care, special attention should be directed to AIDS patients in prisons, families should accept and care for their members who have AIDS, and educational ministries should design programs for prevention.

The United States Catholic Conference

The CCC letter does not discuss condoms or spermicide. The issue of prophylactics is, however, explicitly addressed by the bishops at the national level. In November 1987, the United States Catholic Conference (USCC) published a pastoral letter entitled, *The Many Faces of AIDS: A Gospel Response.* "Because the prospects for the treatment of

---

[7] "Los Angeles Archdiocese" often will be abbreviated as "LAA." See Appendix B for Quick Reference of Abbreviations.

AIDS have been so dismal," note the bishops, "emphasis — and hope — has focused more on its prevention, and this is where the greatest controversy has emerged" (USCC:13).

The bishops emphasize that the Church calls for people to live in "monogamous, heterosexual relationships of lasting fidelity in marriage" (USCC:15). This, they assert, is the solution to the spread of the AIDS virus, and precludes emphasis on condoms and spermicides in AIDS education: "...We oppose the approach to AIDS prevention often popularly called "safe sex" (USCC:16).

This passage, however, is followed by what has become a more controversial one: for those who will not refrain from sexual or intravenous drug-abuse behavior, "educational efforts, if grounded in the broader moral vision outlined above, could include accurate information about prophylactic devices or other practices proposed by some medical experts as potential means of preventing AIDS. We are not promoting the use of prophylactics, but merely providing information that is part of the factual picture" (USCC:18).

When this letter was published, newspaper editors splashed headlines across their front pages heralding the Church's "unprecedented" position on condoms. As one author of the document — Bishop Anthony G. Bosco — explains, "Anytime you have a story that has bishops and condoms in it, you've got a grabber." The USCC statement, says Bishop Bosco, who is Third Bishop of Greensburg, Pennsylvania and a member of the USCC's AIDS Task Force, "is not advocacy [of condoms] — it's information. Many of us felt it would be unrealistic to write a document without even mentioning the "c" word." According to some observers, the excessive media attention forced the Church hierarchy into a corner, compelling, for example, the Los Angeles Archdiocese to publicly dilute the USCC's message.[8] Archbishop Roger Mahony revised the portion of the letter on condoms as follows: "...Recommendation in materials concerning the use of prophylactic devices is not to be endorsed by educators operating under Catholic auspices" (Dart,'87:32).

Several members of the clergy consider the USCC letter too liberal, and its contents were redebated at the USCC's meeting in June, 1988. According to Bishop Bosco, who was present at the meeting, "None of us wanted to see the document withdrawn or repudiated, and it wasn't." Instead, he says, another document will be written in the November 1988, USCC meeting to *complement* — not replace — the first one. For the second document, as one Catholic AIDS activist notes, the question remains, "Will the message be sustained or will it be watered down?"

Catholics Against AIDS: the Praxis

While the Church is still debating what to say, its lower echelons have already plunged into action. According to Church officials, there are an estimated three million Catholics in the Archdiocese of Los Angeles — about fifty percent with Spanish surnames.[9] The Los Angeles Archdiocese, the nation's largest, stretches from Orange County through Santa Barbara, and Pomona to the Pacific Ocean. It encompasses Santa Barbara, Ven-

---

[8] "The media blew it completely out of proportion," recalls Jennie Reyes, a Latina eucharistic minister and AIDS activist. "I mean it was a disaster. I can understand how the Archbishop has had to be very careful."

[9] Some estimate the Latino population to be more than sixty-five percent (see Del Olmo).

tura, and Los Angeles counties. It has the largest concentration of Latino Catholics in the country—an estimated two million (Hernandez, 1986).

There are three realms in which the Archdiocese has responded to the AIDS crisis: spiritual support, practical care, and educational outreach. The issue of morality in AIDS education has compelled the Church to steer initially onto the path of least resistance: ministry to people already affected by the disease. The Church's strongest response, therefore, is in its ministry to people with AIDS (PWAs) and their families and loved ones. "More and more priests are making a foray into the Gay community," says Armando Ochoa, auxiliary bishop of the region of San Fernando. "It's very challenging—on the fringe of the North Hollywood area some priests are working full time with Gays and Lesbians."

For clergy providing spiritual care and counseling to people with AIDS, Church doctrine on homosexuality appears to present less of an obstacle than one might expect. The Church distinguishes between "sexual orientation" and "sexual practice." One Los Angeles clergyman explains, "In our teaching, it's all right for someone to be Gay." The problem arises, he says, in the homosexual act. "One could not couple with another and still be accepted by the Church. It doesn't matter how meaningful the relationship is—that's where our doctrine draws the line. Homosexuals have to be celibate. That's been the traditional teaching through the centuries." The Church encourages homosexuals to channel their sexuality into prayer, ministry, involvement in parish activities, and community service. Explains Bishop Ochoa, "Our alternative is to deal with them as any other person, Gay or straight...to really incorporate them into the life activity of the parish."

In October 1986, Archbishop Roger Mahony established the Office of Pastoral Ministry to Persons with AIDS and to the Lesbian and Gay community. Its director, Father Brad Dusak, in residence at St. Matthew's Parish in Long Beach, recruited priests from the Archdiocese to participate in the program. Approximately 140 priests are now available to volunteer spiritual and religious counseling to people with HIV infection, ARC, or AIDS, and to their families and friends. The Catholic priests are the largest component connected to the AIDS Pastoral Care Network, an interdenominational referral resource coordinated by APLA's[10] Office of Religious Resources.

In April, 1988, the Archbishop commissioned forty priests (gave them a special assignment to work with people with AIDS). The ceremony took place in Blessed Sacrament Church in Hollywood and, according to one observer, the meeting of AIDS patients and priests on the altar was characterized by many "hugs and tears."

According to Father Brad Dusak, AIDS ministry ranges from simply "touching" and "listening" to the person, to "helping the person with AIDS come to terms with the initial shock of a positive diagnosis" and "helping the person and his family get back together" (Dellinger:3).

Pastoral care is one important way the Church can employ its spiritual authority to prevent families and friends from ostracizing people with AIDS. Not only does this alleviate some of the psychological pain and loneliness suffered by the patients, but it helps to relieve the pressure on hospitals and public resources for their care. To instill compassion into the friends and families of AIDS patients is one of the missions outlined in the CCC's *A Call to Compassion:* "Reminding them of our ministry that human dignity comes from God, and that we believe each person is sacred—a unique reflection of God among us—we can encourage them to accept these persons with AIDS back within their

---

[10] AIDS Project Los Angeles.

embrace. Other families might find the courage and strength to provide care in their homes for those incapacitated by AIDS" (CCC:3).

Encouraging families who are not related to AIDS patients to provide care for them will be one of the objectives of several hospices being planned by the Archdiocese. Under the direction of Peter McDermott, the Archdiocese has established the Serra Ancillary Care Corporation, which will oversee four residences for people with AIDS. The first residence opened in July 1988 in a Los Angeles neighborhood of mixed ethnicity (Latino, Black and Asian). Volunteers will be drawn from the surrounding communities to work in the homes, which will provide a place to stay for patients, regardless of ability to pay. It is hoped that families will be found to take patients into their homes and care for them there.

Meanwhile, Father Matt O'Connor, a Dominican from the Southern Province, has established a program that targets homeless AIDS patients. "There are a number of people who aren't in our health system and fall through the cracks," he notes. To serve this clientele, O'Connor is working with the AIDS Interfaith Council to establish a hospice.

That Church doctrine essentially requires Gays to deny their sexuality and lead priestly lives has been rejected by many Catholics. Explains one clergyman, "Some in the Church, like Father Curran, would say the truly Gay person — man or woman — for the sake of completion, for the sake of community. . .should be allowed some kind of union. He would go on to say it should be a stable, monogamous relationship."

An independent Catholic group in Los Angeles advocates the viability of such an alternative lifestyle within the Church. Called Dignity, it is a chapter of the twenty-year-old national organization founded in New York. According to Rafael Vega, president of the Hollywood organization of Catholic Gays and Lesbians, most of the members of Dignity probably haven't stopped going to their own parish churches, but they come to Dignity for support. Although Dignity is not permitted to use Church facilities for services, every Sunday Catholic priests come to Dignity to say mass.

The realm of response to the AIDS crisis in which the Los Angeles Archdiocese has most dragged its feet is education. As one Catholic clergyman involved in AIDS education comments, "I think education to avoid getting the disease is something the Church is struggling with, perhaps we'd have to say too slowly. . . .It's not an easy issue."

At present, the Catholic school system of the Los Angeles Archdiocese, consisting of 228 elementary and fifty-eight secondary schools, has no official AIDS education directives or curricula. According to the Archdiocese, individual schools are depending on the "imagination and creativity" of their teachers and administrators. The diocese of San Jose — "probably the most progressive diocese outside of San Francisco, sensitive to the Gay lifestyle," according to one Los Angeles priest — has developed a resource paper on AIDS which has been distributed to all the schools in the Los Angeles Archdiocese. The Archdiocese is waiting for the National Catholic Education Association to publish its proposed AIDS program, while the Association in turn is waiting for the USCC to clarify its position on prophylactics.

Eighty-five of the 230 Catholic elementary schools in the Archdiocese are connected to its Instructional Television Station. Only those parishes able to afford it are connected, however, and Latino communities, which tend to be poorer, are underrepresented in this system. An AIDS video has yet to be produced by the station. One that was to be strictly about the pastoral aspect of AIDS care was started and then dropped due to a conflict with the hospice in Long Beach that was to be featured in the program. According to Sister Jeanne Harris of the Communications Department, "Our efforts have been put on hold."

The television station and other communications resources of the Church may become more directed toward Latino communities when the Archdiocese completes a media study it has commissioned. The study, to cost more than $50,000, will employ a phone survey to examine the needs and media practices of Latino audiences.

Programs similar to those in the Los Angeles Archdiocese are underway in many of the approximately 500 dioceses and archdioceses across the nation. In New York, for instance, the Archdiocese is opening residences, such as Mother Teresa's in Greenwich Village, for people with AIDS. According to Director of Health and Hospitals Monsignor James P. Cassidy, the archdiocesan hospitals have one-third to one-half of the AIDS patients in the city, and the largest special unit on AIDS in the country.

In Chicago the Archdiocese is launching programs for emergency services for AIDS patients, such as the provision of food, shelter, and clothing. The Alexian Brothers are opening a residence called the Bonaventure House in August 1988. Five Chicago parishes have formed a coalition to address the issue of AIDS. According to Marianne Zelewsky, coordinator for the AIDS ministry for the Chicago Archdiocese, for the fall of 1988 "there's a very comprehensive educational program in place," including AIDS education sermons and meetings with parents in all of the parishes.

In San Francisco, the Archdiocese has been using a hotel as a residence for homeless AIDS patients. Its own thirty-two-room facility is scheduled to open in August 1988. In addition, Mother Teresa's Missionaries of Charity will be opening residences for people with AIDS. The San Francisco Church has also designed an educational outreach program focusing on the "psycho-spiritual" aspects of the disease. Aimed toward AIDS patients, their loved ones, caregivers (such as nurses and social workers), and the general populace, the program focuses exclusively on how people come to grips—psychologically and spiritually—with AIDS, and is meant to complement educational programs aimed at understanding and prevention.

These nationwide efforts, as well as the bishops' letters, are evidence that in Catholic circles AIDS is an increasingly active issue: Catholics are talking about AIDS. "Our priests are constantly being encouraged to update themselves on the AIDS crisis," notes Bishop Ochoa about the Los Angeles Archdiocese. Father Brad Dusak and Father Peter Liuzzi (director of religious formation at Carmel West Seminary) hold medical and theological orientation sessions about AIDS for clergy in the five regions of the Los Angeles Archdiocese. "Archbishop Mahony is calling priests to minister to people with AIDS," says Father Liuzzi. "I think that says a lot to our people." Liuzzi lectured on AIDS to 850 people in March 1988 at the Religious Education Congress, an annual Diocesan event primarily for Catholic teachers.

Catholic laity play a crucial role in generating discourse on the issue. For example, Jennie Reyes, who is mourning the recent loss of her son to AIDS, provides educational workshops in Los Angeles not only to Catholic clergy but to people of other faiths as well. A eucharistic minister in what she describes as a "very conservative" parish, Reyes finds the Church open to learning about and discussing AIDS. "The Church definitely does care," she says. "They want to help."

Reyes belongs to the AIDS Interfaith Council of Los Angeles, and was just recently elected to its new, Washington-based national board on which she is the only Latino representative. She describes the recent meeting in Washington: "In this gigantic room we had laity and clergy together and we had many different faiths together. It was very powerful—we've come together as one big church to address the AIDS crisis."

Drawing from her personal experience of being Latina, having a leadership role in the Church, being divorced, struggling with single parenthood, and facing the reality of AIDS in her own family, Reyes has become a prominent media figure. She has produced television spots with the CDC, and her picture and a quote is in the U.S. Department of Health and Human Services' Spanish brochure, "Entendiendo el SIDA (AIDS)."[11] Reyes, who has organized a support group for mothers of people with AIDS, thinks the Church is essential for AIDS education in the Latino community: "It's a big job for the Church, but I feel the only way the Latinos can be reached is through the Church."

On the national level, in October 1986 the Catholic Church joined members of the religious press in Washington, D.C. for a conference organized by the CDC, the Associated Church Press, and the National Leadership Coalition on AIDS (of which the Catholic Health Association is a member). Entitled, "AIDS: the Challenge to Organized Religion," the conference was designed for religious writers to discuss their response to the disease.

"...Our religious, cultural, and personal presuppositions stared us in the face as we attempted to *talk* about how to *write* about AIDS, relates one Christian writer. "Like the secular press, the religious press has offered too little too late....We cannot love God without loving our neighbor, and right now our neighbor has AIDS" (Seibert:260).

Meanwhile, the Catholic Health Association convened a group of experts in early January 1988 to form an advisory panel for its AIDS programs. "Participants included advocates, administrators, health care providers, religious,[12] and clergy," reports *Catholic Health World*. "The group was asked to 'blue sky' about their own frustrations and unmet needs in dealing with AIDS. Within the first hour, participants identified seventy-seven issues that need attention." One of those issues was a "crying need" for education among members of the religious community. "The role of the Church in helping persons with AIDS with their spiritual needs could be enormous," participants said.

The National Catholic Education Association held a convention during Easter week, 1988, in which it designed a curriculum for AIDS education in Catholic schools. Its proposal is being withheld, however, until the USCC clarifies its official position on prophylactics.

Then, in May 1988, a conference called "AIDS: Religious Respond" was held in Georgetown (Washington,D.C.). It focused on the implications of AIDS for ministry and the concerns of Catholic religious. This conference was followed by the National Catholic AIDS Ministry Conference in June 1988, which took place at the University of Notre Dame in Indiana. Twenty different Catholic communities from around the nation sponsored the conference (primarily orchestrated by the Franciscan Lazzaro Center in New York), which featured workshops on such subjects as the medical aspects of AIDS, pastoral care for persons with AIDS, and building an educational curriculum. A special track program in the conference was reserved for pastoral issues in the care of AIDS patients who are minorities, although no special slot was reserved for focus on the Latino population.

---

[11] Translated as "Understanding AIDS," this brochure was sent to Spanish-speaking homes in the United States. An English version was sent to the rest of America.

[12] "Religious" in this sense is a noun referring to Catholic nuns and brothers.

The Latino Question

While the programs of the Los Angeles Archdiocese appear promising, their commitment to target the Latino population remains elusive. The Latino community has sounded the alarm: "...Experts fear that a catastrophic AIDS outbreak within the substantial L.A. Latino community — whose more than two million residents represent nearly one-third of the area's total population — may be unavoidable unless education efforts are drastically increased," writes Ruben Martinez, Latin Affairs Editor of the *L.A. Weekly* (Martinez,1987). Church workers, meanwhile, are also aware of the problem. "Hispanics are influenced by the Church and by their own culture," reflects one Catholic AIDS activist. "There is a very strong denial that goes on about the whole issue of homosexuality. The whole macho culture precludes anyone from accepting and dealing with it. The Church needs to address the issue. Since they are influential in that community, they must lead the way." Yet while all of the AIDS programs of the Los Angeles Archdiocese certainly include Latinos, a special effort for the Latino population — from the higher echelons of the Church — is strangely absent.

This is especially curious given that one of Archbishop Mahony's objectives since assuming office in September 1985 has been to increase activism of the Church in Latino communities. In May 1986 he launched a program of social activism for the Latino community. Called the "Plan for Hispanic Ministry," its aim is to "restore, strengthen and deepen" Latino faith in the Church. An unprecedented crowd of Latinos — nearly 50,000 — attended the festivities in Dodger Stadium that introduced the plan (Chandler,1986).

The lack of official directives to target the Latino community in the Archdiocese mirrors a similar void in the USCC and CCC pastoral letters. In the California Bishop's letter, there is no mention of the heavy burden of AIDS on Latino communities — nor of their special educational and pastoral needs.

The national Bishop's Conference letter, conversely, does provide special attention to the plight of Latinos, albeit in a footnote. "One of the most sensitive issues faced in the preparation of this statement," the note reads, "is the fact that disproportionate numbers of Blacks and Hispanics have been infected by the AIDS virus. Raising this issue could be perceived as motivated by racism, which is contrary to the very gospel spirit that informs this statement. On the other hand, to ignore the pertinent statistics could contribute to the spread of the disease among some of the most vulnerable and marginalized members of our society" (USCC:8). This statement is followed by statistics about the prevalence of AIDS among minorities.

That the fear of stigmatizing minorities is responsible for the Church hierarchy's silence on the Latino issue is underscored by Father Thomas Gallagher, secretary of education for the USCC, who participated in the USCC meeting: "In the initial discussion, [racism] was an issue that surfaced. People were talking about how Haitians were stigmatized in the early stage. Rather than focus too much on [minority populations], we let the statistics speak for themselves, and that carries with it concern for these populations."

While Church workers acknowledge there is a need for special attention to the Latino situation, they are vague about how that need is being addressed. Weak statements like "I don't think much has been done in that area," "I don't think we've gone that far to make it a special project," and "On those Hispanics we come into contact with, I think we'd be able to have an effect," are common. Some priests, like Father Edward Barrett, Roman Catholic chaplain at the West L.A. Veterans Administration Hospital and an active volunteer in APLA, recognize there is a dearth of activity: "The Church has been very behind, especially for the Hispanics."

As the following discussion of linkages reveals, this lack of attention to the special plight of the Latino population is in part due to the paucity of cooperative efforts launched between the Church and nonsectarian institutions.

LINKAGES

Since our resources for combatting the AIDS epidemic are limited, cooperation among government agencies, private organizations, and religious institutions is crucial. For the Latino community, what linkages have been established between the Catholic Church and nonsectarian AIDS programs? Do AIDS activists recognize the potential of the Catholic Church? What are the obstacles—real and perceived—to establishing cooperative efforts?

The Catholic Church is at once a monolithic "empire" and a conglomeration of little, independent "states." As Sister Jeanne Harris of the Los Angeles Archdiocese Department of Telecommunications suggests, "It's a very strange animal. Sometimes never the two shall meet. It's a grace and a detriment—we could get a lot more done, and yet we wouldn't have the freedom."

Today's Catholic Church is by definition a delicate balance between the theocratic rule of the Vatican and the autonomous action of local parishes. Its very existence is at once harmonic and dissonant. The experience of liberation theology, especially in Latin America, testifies to the tension between the theoretical interpretations of the Bible by the Vatican and the practical interpretations of the meaning of Christianity emerging from grassroots experience. On the parish level, theological orientations of priests, nuns, brothers, and laity often assume a radical character as they interpret Christ's teachings in light of the concrete situation of their parishioners.[13] The Church, although not compelled to advertize the fact, is internally polarized by its conservative and liberal factions. Simplistically categorized, a cleavage has formed between the "Church hierarchy" and the "liberation theologians," or the "Church establishment" and the "Church of the people."

With such a polarization, one can expect wide variations in the approach of individual parishes to the AIDS crisis. It is perhaps in the local, grassroots context that linkages between the Church and nonsectarian organizations are most promising. As one Latino community worker observes on the issue of AIDS, "I don't think it's going to be the whole Church that's going to come around. It's going to be the individual parishes."

In the realm of physical, psychological, and spiritual care for people already affected by the disease, the linkages between the Church and AIDS organizations appear strongest. The Los Angeles Archdiocese's Serra Ancillary Care Corporation, for in-

---

[13] An example is the concept of "sin." Liberation theologians protest the Church's traditional obsession with individual sin, such as stealing and sex outside of marriage, and its nescience of the powerful—and more insidious—"corporate sin" that causes the social and environmental ills of hunger, oppressive human relations, and pollution.

stance, is getting "great reception" from state agencies such as the Health Department, according to Sister Jane Francis Power, director of the Department of Health Affairs of the Archdiocese. Funds have been earmarked for the program by the County and the City of Los Angeles. The residences for people with AIDS, designed to rely heavily on volunteers, will facilitate links with nonsectarian organizations. "Although we haven't developed some of those ties," says Peter McDermott, the Serra Ancillary Care Corporation's director, "I think we'll be looking for them in groups like El Centro."[14]

A leader in forging ties with the Catholic Church — both in the care of AIDS patients and in preventive education — is AIDS Project L.A. (APLA), a large and private nonprofit organization that provides support services for people with AIDS and AIDS education programs to professionals and the public. APLA coordinates the AIDS Pastoral Care Network, an interdenominational referral service for AIDS patients, their families, and loved ones needing spiritual support, in which the Catholic contingent is the largest. "We keep a very close working relationship with the Catholic Church," says United Methodist Reverend Thomas Reinhart-Marean, administrator of the program. Priests are also on APLA's Speakers Bureau, and the organization has cooperated with the Church on several occasions in providing AIDS education.

The extent to which APLA's Church linkages are directed by the institution toward Latinos, however, is questionable. In July 1988, three Latino AIDS workers resigned from APLA in protest over its lack of sensitivity to minority needs. Two of the employees who resigned, Daniel Lara and Zoila Escobar, were the same individuals largely responsible for nurturing linkages with the Church. Church linkages in the interest of the Latino community thus appear to have been largely an individual, rather than institutionalized, effort.

The biggest perceived obstacle to Church/nonsectarian collaboration in the educational arena is the issue of prophylactics. Theoretically, the disagreement between the Church and other institutions over emphasis on condoms creates an insurmountable barrier between the two. The reality, however, is quite different. There is evidence of truth in one observer's comment that it is the media's focus on condoms that compels the Church to be "more repressive in public than in private."

It appears that there is a wide spectrum of interpretation of the Church's official position on prophylactics. Views of Church workers vary from "We can, in the case of AIDS education, talk about the use of condoms" to "We can't teach the use of condoms." There have been several instances, meanwhile, of nonsectarian and Church collaboration on AIDS education where the nonsectarian educator has been permitted to discuss condoms; thus the promotion of condom usage, has been allowed on the periphery of the Church's physical and ideological territory.

According to Father Edward Barrett, "No longer is the issue of dealing with condoms an issue." The best prevention method, he says, is still celibacy, but the Church is beginning to realize that many people will not abstain. (Barrett has given AIDS lectures to unwed pregnant young women at St. Ann's Maternity Hospital. The number of Catholic high school girls impregnated, he notes, is about the same as that of non-Catholic school girls.) "The educational programs now will be much more direct. How direct, I don't know."

---

[14] "El Centro," or "The Center," is a mental health and social work training center for Latinos. It coordinates the Milagro AIDS Project.

An example of the peripheral teachings about condoms is in the lectures Father Barrett has given with APLA personnel at Catholic High schools: he didn't speak of condoms, but the APLA worker did.

Zoila Escobar, former bilingual health educator and outreach worker with the Latino community for APLA (and one of the Latino staff members who resigned from the organization), has provided one-hour presentations on AIDS to several parishes and Catholic schools. Her presentation, she notes, doesn't change much in or out of Church. "We may talk about condoms as long as we talk about the other side of the coin."

For Escobar, in AIDS education there is no separation between Latinos and their faith. "This is a very spiritual community and we have to deal with that," she says. "Because I'm working with Latinos, I always have to address the religious issue whether I'm in the Church or not. . . . We use [the Church] to get into or out of an issue. . . . The Church plays a very important role in our lives."

The Milagro AIDS Project, run by the organization El Centro, is another leader in establishing linkages with the Catholic Church in the realm of AIDS education. Raquel Salinas, who leads "platicas" (informal talks) about AIDS with Spanish-speaking teachers, parents, and students, gave her presentation to a biology class in a Catholic high school. "There were two priests in the audience, and they were very receptive. They liked my style," recalls Salinas, who as part of the presentation demonstrates the use of a condom over her finger. Salinas has been invited by the high school for more presentations.

The Milagro AIDS Project was one of the groups participating in the AIDS education masses, organized by APLA staff, at Our Lady Queen of Angels Church on Memorial Day weekend. That event, in which nonsectarian organizations distributed their AIDS education information on the church steps, is another example of the Church tolerating the promotion of prophylactics on its periphery.

It is crucial to remember, meanwhile, that the promotion of prophylactics as a means of protection is only one facet of AIDS education. Latino writers have suggested that Latinos are five years behind the rest of the country in their basic awareness of the disease.[15] A major step in AIDS education for Latinos, therefore, is the simple act of getting people to talk about the biological realities of the disease.

Since nonsectarian institutions promote the use of condoms in their educational materials, however, the Church cannot make use of such materials. In this light, Father Lawrence Caruso, associate superintendent of the Los Angeles Archdiocese Catholic Schools (where he estimates forty percent of the students are Latino), explains the lack of cooperativism between public and Catholic schools: "No, we haven't [established linkages] to be very honest. First of all, we have not been invited. But we also come from a different point of view, especially with. . .the use of condoms. . . . Our problem is that we can't teach the use of condoms. . . . You can teach statistical facts on it, but you can't teach it as a suitable means because it's not part of our teachings." The Catholic school system does, however, use materials published by the Red Cross: "We use everything they have except the part on condoms."

One of several organizations responsible for targeting the Latino communities nationwide is Sosa and Associates, a Latino marketing agency in San Antonio, Texas. Lily Bendaña, coordinator of the AIDS education project begun in August 1987, says the goal of the first phase of the education campaign (for which Sosa and Associates was sub-

---

[15] See *Preciado*, 1988.

contracted by Ogilvy and Mather Public Affairs, whose AIDS program is in turn funded by the CDC) was to simply introduce to the Latino community the fact that AIDS is a serious problem. The second phase of the program targets the sexually active woman in and outside of marriage.

In both phases, part of their advertising campaigns have been directed toward the Catholic Church. According to Bendaña, "The Catholic Church, which is the most influential of the churches among Hispanics, is very compassionate. . . .If the materials in any way talk about condoms, they won't use them. To the Church, that is not an option. There's no question — they have been very clear about that." Yet Bendaña considers the issue of morality with the Church no obstacle: "They help us a lot. Just by getting people out to talk about AIDS — that's a huge undertaking. We would love to see [them say], for example, 'Yes, if you cannot abstain, use condoms,' but [their stance] is not an obstacle. Our goal is to educate people on how you get AIDS and how you can't get it."

Bendaña also points out that the U.S. Department of Health guidelines and the Church's teachings are largely congruent: "The number one prevention tool is abstinence and monogamy. The number *two* prevention tool is 'O.K., If you cannot do these things, then condoms are the next best thing.'"

The congruencies between Church and nonsectarian objectives in AIDS education are underscored by the experience of Father Gallagher of the USCC, who is serving on a panel with the Educational Development Center (EDC) of Boston. The panel is designing an AIDS education package for the EDC curriculum.

When one proposed text was presented at a meeting, he recalls, "before I had a chance to say anything, everyone else beat it up. They said the part about condoms didn't have enough caution on the risks involved even [with their protection]. People were referring to *The Many Faces of AIDS*[16] in their interventions about the text." The nonsectarian educators, in other words, paralleled the Church in their concern that AIDS education go beyond simply "getting them down to the drug store" to buy condoms.

Additional forms of collaboration are occurring on the national level. Professionals from outside the Church hierarchy presented papers at the National Catholic AIDS Ministry Conference at Notre Dame in late June 1988. Among those presenting was Lou Tesconi, the lawyer who, six weeks after beginning studies for priesthood, was expelled from his seminary for having been diagnosed with AIDS.[17] His workshop concerned models of ministry within the Church for persons with AIDS.

Reverend Reinhart-Marean of the APLA Pastoral Care Network agrees that the Church's moral stance is not as much of an obstacle to collaboration as one might expect. Many of APLA's educational materials, he notes, are distributed during speaking engagements in the parishes.

Yet the fact remains that the Church is restricted by its position in the extent to which it can utilize pamphlets, posters, video and audio programs, and other types of handouts produced by nonsectarian institutions. As Sister Jeanne Harris of the Los Angeles Archdiocese Telecommunications Office notes, "We cannot use most of the stuff being put out by most of the producers because they all get into the condom thing."

---

[16] The USCC pastoral letter.

[17] Tesconi subsequently created the Damien Ministry, named after a priest who worked with leprosy sufferers and died of the disease.

The existence of these limitations begs the question: should nonsectarian institutions tailor their materials to the needs of the Catholic Church for the sake of multiplying their distribution possibilities and reaching Latinos?

Reverend Reinhart-Marean suggests the task would be too formidable: "The complexity of doing AIDS education within faith communities requires that we do so with extreme sensitivity, with respect for the values of each community we deal with."

The complexity of such a task, however, is debatable. Sister Harris notes, "We've seen some [video programs] that could be used judiciously, maybe by turning them off early." This suggests that only a slight alteration of the program would permit its use by the Church, a strong argument for tailoring productions for the Catholic Church in order to get the basic information about AIDS out.

There are several reasons that linkages between Church and nonsectarian institutions have been nonexistent or are only now germinating. On the one hand, the Church is limited in its collaboration by its position on prophylactics. On the other hand, it appears AIDS activists in nonreligious organizations often perceive such linkages as too difficult to achieve; many of these groups have chosen what they consider the path of least resistance by focusing on other institutions.

"We have too many other avenues we can take," explains one Latino community worker. "Ideally, it would be great. . . .But just trying to get into the [public] schools is difficult. . . .Everyone's afraid of lawsuits." Indeed, AIDS activists are preoccupied with overcoming other obstacles. The L.A. Unified School District has yet to establish a curriculum for AIDS education, and community organizations are having difficulty accessing its students. "We have a problem going into the public schools," notes Michael Puente of the AIDS action organization Cara a Cara.[18] "We have contacts, but the LAUSD[19] is extremely conservative. It's very difficult for us to give presentations on AIDS in the schools."

Another source of sluggishness in establishing linkages is what appears to be an only vague awareness on the part of some AIDS activists of the diversity of individual parishes, their activities around the AIDS issue, and their potential to reach Latinos. One Latino AIDS worker, for instance, when asked about the potential of the Church, replied, "I think it's great, if they would just accept doing the AIDS education. There have been some priests who have been open to working with people with AIDS." Another stated, "You're dealing with direct confrontation when you talk of safe sex or use of condoms."

One reason for the lack of awareness may be that the Church is doing, but not telling. "I have to convince people that the Church is doing things," observes eucharistic minister Jennie Reyes. "People don't know. . .partly because the Church doesn't advertise what they're doing. I don't know [why]. People need to know what the Church is doing."

Zoila Escobar, who while at APLA was "getting all the calls" from the Church for AIDS education because her organization was among the few providing it to the parishes, surmises that people consider the Church inapproachable. "I think a lot of people think that," she says. "I used to think that."

Some Latino community workers, meanwhile, feel the Church has not yet recognized the urgency of the AIDS crisis. "It has not been a priority of ours to work with the

---

[18] Cara a Cara, or "Face to Face," offers AIDS education and prevention, support groups, and testing primarily to monolingual Spanish speakers. The organization is part of the Hollywood Sunset Community Clinic.

[19] The Los Angeles Unified School District.

Church," says one Latino AIDS activist. "The Church has been very slow to act and instead of working with them we're working in spite of them. . . .It's not that there's any animosity."

Resentment, however, does seem to play a role in the dearth of cooperative efforts. Many working on behalf of people affected by AIDS have alternative lifestyles and political perspectives; they resent the Church's rigid doctrine on such universal issues as homosexuality and birth control.

The resentment clearly flows both ways. In an interview with the *National Catholic Reporter,* Archbishop John R. Quinn of San Francisco said in reference to a Gay activist group, "If they would not be attacking the moral teaching of the Church, we could all work together. But they insist on this, and that makes it very difficult" (Dellinger, 1987).

Some AIDS activists suggest Protestant churches are more tolerant of diversity and therefore easier to work with. "[Protestants] are in the twentieth century," says one Latino AIDS worker. "I think the Catholic Church is still in the Seventeenth. . . .We're still fighting for our Mass in Spanish."

THE EFFECT OF AIDS ON THE CHURCH

While much of Church doctrine is indeed centuries old, as liberation theology shows it is not static. This chapter has explored how the Catholic Church can affect the impact of AIDS on the Latino population. Equally important, however, is how the AIDS crisis impacts on the Church itself.

In mobilizing its human and material resources around the AIDS crisis, priests, nuns, brothers, and laity are forced to systematically address the sacred realm of sexuality—publicly, and in graphic, concrete ways. AIDS has forced the Church into a corner, compelling it, for instance, to inform its faithful—as a health measure—about birth control methods to which it is morally opposed.

Father Rodney Demartini, director of AIDS education for the Archdiocese of San Francisco, suggests the social turbulence resulting from AIDS being a sex-related disease is evident in the rest of society as well as in the Church. "It's challenging us—as human beings—at our most vulnerable points."

Church doctrine on homosexuality

One of those vulnerable and controversial areas is homosexuality. Due to the AIDS crisis, for the first time the Church is interacting extensively with the homosexual population. "There has been very little contact between Church people and well-adjusted Gay people," notes Rafael Vega of Dignity. Until the AIDS crisis, most of the Gay people with which the Church came into contact were "disturbed and in confession." Today, however, the Church is ministering to homosexuals whose problem is not their sexuality; rather, it is their loved ones, who have fallen victim to a fatal disease. The Church is helping thousands of Gay people with AIDS and their significant others to cope with a tragedy, and this experience is transforming the face of the Church itself.

"Essentially what's happening is we're going from statistics to faces," says Father Brad Dusak. "As soon as you put faces to something, it's less of a bogeyman." Priests, nuns, brothers, and laypersons are beginning to understand the homosexual experience in a more positive light. "I think it's very true that for many people there is a certain growth in compassion," reflects Raphael Vega. "When you have seen the other suffer and walked with the other in their pain, maybe you begin to appreciate that you were misunderstanding the whole thing."

Health educator Zoila Escobar, who has designed a workshop on sexuality and AIDS education to present to a group of Catholic sisters, is also witnessing this transformation in the Church: "I think the nuns and priests are much more open-minded than we think. I'm finding that out....The Pope can make rules because he is removed. But those priests and nuns who are working with reality, with the people at the grassroots level, are much more understanding of people who are not nuns and priests."

"For a lot of people," notes a priest who cares for AIDS patients on a regular basis, "if they deal with a Gay person, I think what begins to happen is they being to realize there's something going on here besides promiscuity." As the stereotypes about Gay lifestyles begin to dissolve, he suggests, the Church is compelled to look more closely at itself: "Anyone who is involved, seeing things from the inside, begins to agonize themselves over the present teaching of the Church....I believe that's what's going on right now—a development and understanding of Gay and Lesbian life....We're almost being forced to be present, to understand, to hear what people are saying, and when that happens it raises all sorts of questions."

Meanwhile, the Church is also facing the reality of AIDS within its own clergy. At least twenty-four cases of the disease have emerged among priests. "The people who are really out on a limb," says Lou Tesconi, founder of Damien Ministry in Washington, "are the diocesan priests." When they get AIDS, he explains, they are sent out of their parishes and often have no support networks to help them cope with the illness.

Many priests are open about their homosexual orientation and reject the Church's position on homosexuality. In the past twenty years the Church has become more tolerant of Gay priests who, like heterosexual priests, are expected to remain celibate. That homosexuality is an active issue in the Church is evidenced in the controversy over the actions of Seattle's Archbishop Raymond Hunthausen and Father Charles Curran:[20] AIDS is one variable propelling this issue into the forefront.

How will this swell of compassion within the Church inspire its theological debates? In speculating on such a question—and speculation is the limit of this exploration—we must keep in mind the Church's dual personality: the rigid, almost impermeable Vatican on the one hand and the fluid, more world-wise, grassroots parishes on the other. At best, the leap from compassion—whose wellsprings are in the praxis of the grassroots Church—to a reformulation of Church doctrine, is complex.

According to Father John Gigrich, associate pastor at St. Matthews in Washington, D.C. and one of the founders of the group Dignity, while involvement in the AIDS crisis generates empathy for Gay people, it does not necessarily increase acceptance of their lifestyle. The homosexual *act*, explains Father Gigrich, who is coordinator of programs for people with AIDS and the Archbishop's special assistant in ministry to homosexual Catholics, is still banned on the grounds of morality.

---

[20] See Corwin, 1987.

Says Sister Jeanne Harris of the Los Angeles Archdiocese Telecommunications Department, working with homosexual people "makes us conscious, more aware of the human side of it, more ready to discuss the issue, to be somewhat free of uninformed judgments of people — you could say it has a liberating effect.... But the only change, as far as internal to the Church goes, is understanding in a compassionate sense; this is not to be confused with understanding of the homosexual lifestyle.... You're living in a sense their lives, but it doesn't change the way you think — it makes you feel for the people, but not in the sense of conviction."

"One of the things that bothers the hell out of me," says Monsignor James Patrick Cassidy, director of health and hospitals for the New York Archdiocese and chancellor of New York Medical College, "is that homosexuals are using the disease as a way to get people to accept their lifestyle." The Church's involvement with people affected by AIDS, explains the Monsignor, "means compassion for the sinner, but not for the sin."

In the July 1988 National Catholic AIDS Ministry Conference at Notre Dame, this crucial distinction — between homosexual orientation and lifestyle — was attacked for being hypocritical and making God appear "sadistic." The conference speaker was John J. McNeil, author of the forthcoming book, *Taking a Chance on God: Liberating Theology for Gays and Lesbians, Their Lovers, Friends and Families.*[21]

"Gay love came out of the closet with AIDS," says McNeil, a former Jesuit priest who was thrown out of the Catholic order in 1987 for publicizing his opposition to Church doctrine on homosexuality. "People who are dealing with AIDS are dealing with couples, and seeing what a powerful and wholesome love that can be."

Even for Church workers ministering with compassion to Gay AIDS patients, he argues, it's "sheer sadism," to accept the orientation while continuing to reject the act. "If gay orientation is O.K., then that's the way God created them.... If God created someone like that, then God is sadistic. I would much rather have them say the orientation is evil.... That's more consistent to me, then you can reject the whole business." McNeil, now a practicing psychotherapist in New York, is the founder of the original chapter of the group Dignity, in New York. In 1978 he published *The Church and the Homosexual* and was consequently forced by the Vatican, as a punishment, to take a vow of silence. When Cardinal Ratzinger published his letter from Rome in 1987 condemning homosexuality as evil, McNeil broke that vow: he published a revised version of *The Church and the Homosexual,* which includes a chapter on AIDS.

McNeil's hope is for Church doctrine to recognize the viability and naturalness of the homosexual lifestyle. That he was one of the three principal speakers at the Notre Dame conference is evidence that a theological debate over this issue is gaining momentum. "People at the conference were amazingly receptive," says McNeil, about his message.

Indeed, the AIDS crisis has facilitated Catholic debate not only about homosexuality, but sexuality in general. Father Brad Dusak, who also attended the Notre Dame conference, described the event as "fantastic — the ease with which everything was discussed was unprecedented and wouldn't have happened five years ago."

The Church, however, is a long road away from resolving the issue of homosexuality, and on that road are centuries of entrenched convictions about human sexuality. Explains Bishop Bosco of the USCC's AIDS Task Force, "I don't anticipate any change in the Church's teachings because the Church sees the gift of sex as bound up in two realities: love and procreation.... It says you can't be exclusive of one or the other."

---

[21] The book will be published by Beacon Press.

Some speculate that the imperative of procreation in all sexual relations could be discredited with science. Already, the AIDS crisis is leading to more questioning within the Church about the nature of homosexuality. "I would imagine that there would be some evaluation," says Sister Jane Francis Power of the Los Angeles Archdiocese Department of Health Affairs, "not so much in the sexual behavior of homosexuals, but certainly of why there are so many people in that category of orientation, and of whether there is some biological reason for this."

In the past, says Sister Power, who has been in the health field fifty-four years, breakthroughs in science have made changes possible in Church doctrine. For example, the Church once considered intervention in ectopic pregnancies in the fallopian tube — a condition often fatal for the mother if her pregnancy is brought to fruition — tantamount to abortion. When it was determined that the ectopic tube was itself pathological in such cases, the Church changed its position by allowing the removal of the tube. "These are finesses of language," says Sister Power, "but they solved our problem."

The Church's involvement in the AIDS crisis, thus, may make it more prone to seize upon scientific proof of the "normalcy" of homosexuality. But "as long as it's considered an abnormal expression," says Sister Power, "I don't think the Church would approve of it."

Church doctrine on birth control

The AIDS crisis may be propelling another issue into the center of the theological arena: birth control. The Church currently allows couples to use "safe period" and CMBBT[22] methods for family planning, but considers all other methods unnatural. The increase in cases of pediatric AIDS would seem a potential impetus for a more liberal birth control policy.

Many observers feel, however, that at least in the short run there will be no change in Church doctrine concerning birth control — even in light of the tragedy of pediatric AIDS.[23] "The Church doesn't establish its moral teachings for pragmatic reasons," explains Bishop Bosco. If a couple has AIDS and wants to prevent pregnancy, "the teaching of the Church would be...they'd have to use abstinence, safe period or CMBBT as birth control methods."

On the level of action in the grassroots Church, however, change is more likely. Observes Lou Tesconi, "Most priests I know haven't paid attention to the whole birth control thing from the beginning. My general sense is that few of the priests agree with Church doctrine on birth control." On the local level, notes Tesconi, priests counsel their parishioners "in their own way." Dr. Patrick Hughes, director of Pastoral Ministry for the Archdiocese of San Francisco, also suggests there is flexibility about birth control on the parish level: "There is a lot of respect for those who prayerfully reflect on what they think they need to do."

---

[22] Cervical Mucous Basal Body Temperature. This method involves daily monitoring of the body's temperature and cervical mucous consistency, to determine the precise time of ovulation and infertile days in the menstrual cycle.

[23] This observation is based on interviews with Bosco, Demartini, Dusak, Harris, Hughes, Kane, McNeil, Tesconi and Power.

If priests and other Church workers in the thousands of parishes across the United States are changing their views on human sexuality, it is conceivable that some day many of these individuals will move into the higher echelons of the Church hierarchy and be able to affect change from the top down. On the other hand, points out Father Demartini of the San Francisco Archdiocese, in many ways "moving up becomes more restrictive. Those of us who are not hierarchically involved are often in a better position to make change."

If Church doctrine does bend in the AIDS storm, it's likely to be a slow process. "The only way [AIDS] is going to affect it is slowly over the period of many, many years," predicts Tesconi. "Over the course of twenty-five to thirty years you might see some change." What is certain, however, is that the volatile issues concerning human sexuality will not disappear from theological debate. At the May 1988 religious conference in Georgetown, Tesconi observed that a common sentiment among those present was that "the Church has to deal with the sexuality issue in general." McNeil echoes this sentiment: "There is a desperate need for a whole rethinking of sexuality, and AIDS is forcing the whole thing to a boiling point." Whether the pot will boil over remains to be seen.

HIV Testing

While the AIDS crisis stimulates theological debates on human sexuality, the Church is also grappling with issues common to other institutions. At the conference in Georgetown, Tesconi met several priests with AIDS. One big issue for the Church right now, he notes, is HIV testing of candidates for the ministry. "There's an undercurrent that's prominent that wants to test," he says, "but my impression is that it's really connected with another issue, that is the Gay issue."

According to Tesconi, who was rejected by his Carmelite seminary for being HIV-positive, the various religious orders of the Catholic Church are currently debating whether or not to give the HIV test to men when they apply to the seminaries — and some orders have already decided to do so. "A lot of these communities are trying to find a reason to test," says Tesconi, "and they can't find a peg on which to hang their hat." Meanwhile, the kind of discrimination he had to face, says Tesconi, is "receding into the background."

Bishop Bosco notes that "some are talking about [testing in seminaries]. We have a health screen much like anyone else. If we're going to accept a young man into the seminary, we need some idea of his health." He doubts, however, any one perspective will become national Church policy, as entry medical examinations have always been in the domain of the individual seminaries.

Church membership

Another social implication of AIDS in the Catholic community concerns Church membership; will more people, because of their experience with Catholic AIDS ministry, join the Church? "Maybe it's going to have a very positive effect on Church attendance," speculates Hughes of the San Francisco Archdiocese. Hughes points out that when people are dying, they begin to search for more profound meaning in their lives and tend to reflect upon God; they experience more of a need for the Church.

Meanwhile, according to Father Brad Dusak, membership in the Church "is going to become more acceptable among Gay people," many of whom were once Catholic but had to choose between the Church and their sexuality. At the same time, individual parishes will become more receptive to people with homosexual lifestyles. Says Dusak, "Certainly there was a time when the Catholic wouldn't accept Aunt Milly into the household because she was divorced." Like divorce, predicts Dusak, homosexuality may become more familiar in parishes: "I think it's going to shock less and less people."

Opposition

On the other end of the spectrum from those directly affected by AIDS are conservatives in the Church who oppose Church involvement in AIDS ministry or education. Are there any negative political or economic ramifications of the Church's involvement in combatting AIDS? "You see articles written by folks that still see AIDS as a punishment by God," notes Hughes, "but there's not a lot of that. . . .Maybe it even has some financial effect, but it hasn't and won't affect the Church's response, which is to have compassion."

Some conservative elements of the Church, observes Father Gigrich of the Washington Archdiocese, oppose ministry to people with AIDS. Gigrich has been "torn apart" in *The Wanderer,* a conservative Catholic newspaper published in Minnesota, for his work with AIDS and the homosexual community, and has also been the object of attack in paid advertisements. Lou Tesconi, meanwhile, received a phone call in June 1988 from a man in New Haven, Connecticut who was rejected by his parish for having contracted AIDS.

But Gigrich and Tesconi are unconcerned that conservative forces will hamper AIDS ministry. Funding will be unaffected, says Gigrich, because in the Church there is very little money earmarked for AIDS specifically; such monies are drawn from general budgets. Tesconi, whose Damien Ministry depends in part on donations, notices that conservative donors perhaps find psychological relief in giving: "My sense is that people say to themselves, 'I'll be happy to give you money, I don't want to deal with it' — They don't want to go near AIDS." The Damien Ministry, notes Tesconi, has raised large sums in conservative communities such as McLean, Virginia.

According to Monsignor Cassidy of New York, there is little opposition to the Church's participation in AIDS ministry or AIDS education. For AIDS projects in the Archdiocese, he says, there is abundant funding. "Some Catholic doctors are worried about being identified with AIDS patients and we've had to be very firm about this — we've said anyone who does that is out." But few object to AIDS ministry, he says, because "[we're] not approving of the homosexual way of life. I run one residence downtown that gets more donations than you would believe."

Cooperation

According to Dr. Patrick Hughes of the San Francisco Archdiocese, "One of the effects AIDS has had, is it has forced the Church to look at its role in cooperating and collaborating with others in response to this crisis." The efforts of his Archdiocese, Hughes notes, have been characterized by a noticeably "high level of cooperation and understanding with folks who are involved in responding to the AIDS crisis. I think it's brought people together who might not otherwise have been together."

In considering the possible effects of cooperation between the Church and other groups, it is important to note that in the political spectrum many AIDS activists are on the left. Many of the groups with which the Church is establishing ties in the AIDS crisis were formed around special interests and philosophies that are outside of the mainstream; their perceptions of the world are framed with a mosaic of feminist, race, and class analyses. The rights of Gays, workers, minorities, and women are often their creeds.

The Church, meanwhile, has been historically tied with the very social and political constructs that these groups, to varying degrees, are fighting to uproot: sexism, imperialism, elitism, racism, and capitalism. Especially before Vatican II, for instance, the Church was notorious for its complicity with the inequitable land-tenure systems and iron-fisted military regimes of Latin America. Such history is salient for many Latino community workers, who recognize the linkages between the oppression of their people in Latin America and the problems faced by Latinos in the United States.

How will this association with community groups that have progressive political agendas — including radical perspectives on sexuality — affect the Church? In Latin America and, in many cases, in the United States, Church involvement with the poor has sometimes made revolutionaries out of priests; radical interpretations of Christ's teachings often result from intimacy with the problems of the underclass. At the very least, many Church workers will be infused with new ideas; the trajectories of these ideas, one can't predict.

The central point of this exploration of the impact of AIDS on the Church itself — its theological debates, institutional policies, and economic and political health — is simple. Under the rubric of "the social consequences of AIDS" are important transformations in the Roman Catholic Church. That these nascent reforms are circumscribed at the grassroots level suggests Church doctrine on human sexuality will remain intact — but this in no way diminishes the relevance of such changes. Indeed, as the Catholic AIDS activists quoted in this chapter have revealed, the Church in the context of community is often more almighty than canon law. The following section returns to the Latino community, and offers recommendations for more effectively combatting the AIDS epidemic.

CONCLUSIONS AND RECOMMENDATIONS

According to observers in the Latino community, Los Angeles AIDS programs for Latinos — and minorities in general — have been "woefully inadequate" (Martinez, 1987). This chapter has argued that one answer to the problem is that all organizations fighting the AIDS epidemic — Latino and non-Latino — should recognize and tap the power of the Roman Catholic Church. The Church, meanwhile, should specifically target the Latino population and consider collaborative efforts with nonsectarian Latino AIDS projects a priority.

The Church, at least verbally, is committed to the concept of cooperation "...We support collaborative efforts by governmental bodies, health providers, and human service agencies," declares the USCC, "to provide adequate funding and care for persons with AIDS" (USCC,1987:11). In addition, "We pledge that we will work with public, private, and other religious groups to achieve the objectives we outlined earlier" (USCC,1987:23).

In the realm of care for those already affected by the disease, the USCC offers the resources of the Church. "...We encourage the use of church facilities as sites for providing various levels and kinds of care" (USCC,1987:23).

Such commitment is also emphasized, with a conciliatory tone, in the realm of AIDS education:

> We also wish to assure legislators and public officials that we are willing to collaborate with them in the development of an informed and enlightened public policy for the prevention of AIDS. (USCC:20).

> ...We recognize that this raises important questions because of existing constitutional restraints or interpretations of the separation of Church and State. We are willing to join other people of good will in dialogue about how...a fuller understanding of human sexuality might be communicated in our public schools and elsewhere. (USCC, 1987:17).

The USCC supports the concept of AIDS education:

> We will also support legislation and educational programs that seek to provide accurate information about AIDS....Pertinent biological data and basic information about the nature of the disease are essential for understanding the biological and pathological consequences of one's personal choices, both to oneself and others. (USCC, 1987:16).

The approaches of the Church and nonsectarian institutions are largely compatible. "Most of AIDS-prevention education is not controversial," points out William Wood, executive director of the CCC in Sacramento. "The information that needs to be communicated has to do with the nature of the disease and how that disease is transmitted (Wood, 1987:399). Church youth groups, organizations, schools, and media outlets can make use of most information on AIDS; the problem lies in separating that information from the promotion of prophylactics.

The Church's moral framework for AIDS education, meanwhile, is less of an obstacle to collaboration than one would expect. Safe sex guidelines, suggests Eunice Diaz, director of Community Affairs at the Seventh Day Adventist White Memorial Center, can be disseminated from many sources other than the Church: "I don't think we have to preach safe sex guidelines from all pulpits."

As Father Peter Liuzzi noted in his address to participants in the AIDS workshop held at the Religious Education Congress, "Abstinence is not the primary response to AIDS on the part of our bishops. If it were...then our bishops would indeed be justly judged as unfeeling and ruthless, much like the disease they are fighting. Examine the Californian bishops' pastoral. You will notice, that after speaking of abstinence, they quickly move on to compassion as the chief response to AIDS..." (Liuzzi,1988:2).

It is clear that cooperative efforts between the Church and nonsectarian organizations depend on compromise from both sides. Instead of insisting that the Catholic

Church change, urges Diaz, organizations should recognize the things for which that institution is best suited: "Use various institutions for the various, multifaceted jobs they can do. . . .People aren't recognizing that the Church is willing and ready to do many, many forms of complimentary social services. Rather than try to change the Church, use it as a mechanism of the social support system."

Organizations working with the crisis of AIDS in the Latino community should use national and local Catholic media outlets for AIDS education. If necessary, they may tailor their message to the moral guidelines of the Church in the interest of disseminating basic information about the disease to as wide an audience as possible, as quickly as possible. They can use other avenues for the promotion of safe sex guidelines.

Nonsectarian organizations must also recognize that the Church is not a homogenous institution, and that some Church workers are more receptive to collaboration than others. Through its ministry to people with AIDS, their families, and their loved ones, the Church itself is undergoing a transformation: its stereotypes of the Gay community are rapidly breaking down.

While Latino organizations must "harness" the Church as one would an energy resource, the Church should in turn launch an effort to directly address the special needs of the Latino population in the AIDS crisis. As Father Luis Olivares of the Los Angeles Archdiocese's largest Latino parish[24] notes, "In the not too distant future, Latinos will be the majority in Catholic Church membership in this country" (Olivares). This fact illustrates that the Church is in an exceptionally advantageous position to become a leader in Latino AIDS education. In the Church, forging ties with Latino AIDS activists should be an urgent priority.

The Latino community, meanwhile, can be instrumental in educating the clergy about AIDS. The Latino Catholic lay person is especially important in this light. "The laity is the Church now," says Jennie Reyes. "As far as their providing leadership is concerned, I as a mother of a person with AIDS have contributed a lot to the knowledge of the Church that they were unaware of."

At the same time, researchers concerned with AIDS policy, and the social consequences of AIDS, should recognize the important role of religion: its effects on attitudes about the epidemic and its potential as a resource for educational outreach and care for those affected. The CDC is funding several national prevention and control programs which require targeting Latino and Black populations. In August 1988, the CDC sponsored a national conference in Washington dedicated to minority outreach, and several Catholic figures and organizations were sent invitations. Research is necessary on how these programs and conferences are tapping resources of the Catholic Church and other religious institutions. Protestant churches are also active in the fight against AIDS; the nature of their programs and linkages with other institutions are worthy of exploration.[25]

The aim of this chapter has been to explore one avenue of hope for the Latino population in the AIDS crisis. Many practical realities in the day-to-day work of AIDS activists have no doubt been ignored in this analysis because they are beyond the experience of the author. Hopefully, Church and nonsectarian workers in the Latino community struggling against the overwhelming tragedy of AIDS can nevertheless find inspiration in this "bird's-eye" view.

---

[24] "La Placita" Our Lady Queen of Angels, in East Los Angeles.

[25] See, for example, Schaper (1987) for Evangelical Lutheran perspective on pastoral care for persons with AIDS and their families, and Mumper (1988) for missionary approach to AIDS in Africa.

Appendix A

Latinos and AIDS

Of all the pediatric AIDS cases, ninety percent are Black and Latino (Mason,1988). According to the Centers for Disease Control in Atlanta, "The incidence of AIDS is rising for all racial/ethnic groups, and in all geographic regions of the country. However, cumulative incidences of AIDS among Blacks and Hispanics are over three times the rate for Whites" (CDC,1986). Education programs to prevent transmission of the virus, according to the CDC, "need to consider that approximately seventy-five percent of heterosexual patients, seventy-three percent of women with AIDS, and ninety-two percent of children with perinatally acquired infection are Black or Hispanic" (CDC, 1986).

A higher percentage of heterosexual adult males in the Latino population is contracting AIDS; nearly half of Latino people with AIDS are heterosexual, while less than fifteen percent of White victims are heterosexual. This has particular ramifications for minority women, since it is easier to transmit the disease from man to woman than vice versa. Latinos comprise about eight percent of the mainland U.S. population but represent fourteen percent of known AIDS cases. "Health officials predict a seven-fold increase in Hispanic AIDS cases over the next four years..." (Preciado,88:8). Twenty-two percent of the 350 children under fifteen who have AIDS are Latino. (All of the statistics in this paragraph are from *Preciado,* 88).

Latino women have an incidence of AIDS eleven times greater than White women. Since 1980, of all Latino AIDS deaths, thirteen percent have been women (Worth and Rodriguez,1987:5). According to Worth and Rodriguez, "The Latina women most at risk are young (one-third of the U.S. Latino population is under fifteen, the median age is twenty-three), poor (forty percent of Latino families are female-headed, 51.3 percent of these below the poverty line), and have little education" (Worth and Rodriguez,1987:6).

Between June 1981 and September 1986, Blacks and Latinos accounted for twenty-three percent and fourteen percent respectively of the 22,468 male AIDS victims. Among women, however, Blacks and Latinos accounted for fifty-one percent and twenty-one percent respectively, out of the 1,634 female cases (CDC,1986). According to the Centers for Disease Control, "Ninety percent of the children with perinatally-acquired AIDS compared with forty-two percent of the children with hemophilia — or transfusion-associated AIDS — were Black or Hispanic" (CDC, 1986).

According to the Centers for Disease control, by March 1988, fourteen percent of all adult and adolescent AIDS cases were Latino (CDC, 1988). Fourteen percent of all children's AIDS cases were also Latino (CDC, 1988).

Appendix B

Quick Reference of Abbreviations

APLA — AIDS Project Los Angeles

CCC — California Catholic Conference

CDC — Centers for Disease Control

PWAs — People with AIDS

USCC — United States Catholic Conference

Bibliography

1. AIDS Ministry, Center for Continuing Education, "National Catholic AIDS Ministry Conference" (Program), Notre Dame, IN 46556.
2. Boodman, Sandra G. "Hispanic Culture Redefines AIDS Fight," *The Washington Post* Mon., Dec. 28, 1987 p. A1
3. CCC (California Catholic Conference). "A Call to Compassion: Pastoral Letter on AIDS to the Catholic Community of California" *Commentary* Vol. VIII, No. 4 (May, 1987), Sacramento, CA.
4. Corwin, Miles. "Gay Priests: A Dilemma for Catholics," *L.A. Times,* Mon., Feb.16, 1987, Front page.
5. Dart, John. "L.A. Archdiocese Revises Statement on AIDS, Condoms," *Los Angeles Times,* Tues., Dec. 22, 1987.
6. Del Olmo, Frank. "Latino Community, with Church's Help, is on Move," (editorial), *L.A. Times,* Thurs., Jun. 12, 1986, Sec.II, p.7.
7. Dellinger, R.W., "AIDS: The Church Responds with Care," *The Tidings* (Los Angeles Diocese Publication) May 1, 1987, p. 3.
8. CDC (Centers for Disease Control). "Acquired Immunodeficiency Syndrome (AIDS) among Blacks and Hispanics — United States," Reprinted by the U.S. Dept. of Health and Human Services, Public Health Service, from MMWR, Oct. 24, Vol 35, No.42, pp. 656–658, 663–666.
9. CDC (Centers for Disease Control). "AIDS Weekly Surveillance Report," United States AIDS Program, Center for Infectious Diseases, May 2, 1988.

10. CHA (Catholic Health Association of the United States). "Meeting at CHA: AIDS Leaders Describe Anguish, Frustration," *Catholic Health World*, Vol.4, No.2 (Jan.15), 1988, p. 1.

11. Chandler, Russel. "Mahony Unveils Broad Latino Aid Plan," *L.A. Times*, Wed., May 28, 1986, Sec. I, p. 11.

12. Duncan, Muriel. "AIDS Crisis: A Challenge to be the Church in Deed and in Truth," *United Church Observer*, January, 1988., pp. 24–33.

13. Editorial, "The AIDS Pandemic and the Church," *Communique*, Nov., 1987.

14. Gallup Poll. August, 1987.

15. Hernandez, Marita. "Celebracion '86" – A Latino Gathering," *L.A. Times*, Sat., May 31,1986, Sec.II., p.4.

16. Hopkins, Donald R. "AIDS in Minority Populations in the United States," *Public Health Reports: Journal of U.S. Public Health Service*, Nov.–Dec., 1987.

17. Liuzzi, Peter J. Address at the AIDS workshop, Religious Education Congress, March, 1988.

18. Martinez, Ruben. "A Death in the Family," *L.A. Weekly*, March 4–10, 1988, p. 25.

19. Martinez, Ruben. "AIDS: The Crisis in Latino L.A.," *L.A. Weekly*, Oct.30–Nov. 5, 1987, p. 10.

20. Martinez, Ruben. "AIDS in the Latino Community," *Americas 2001*, 1987.

21. Mason, James O., M.D., Dr.P.H. (Assistant Surgeon General), "National Conference on the Prevention of HIV Infection and AIDS Among Racial and Ethnic Minorities in the United States," (brochure on August 15–17, 1988 conference). CDC AIDS Conference Office of c/o Associate Consultants, Washington, D.C., June, 1988.

22. Medina, Carmen. *SIECAS Report*, Vol. XV., No.3, January–February, 1987. Sex Information and Education Council of the U.S.

23. Mumper, Sharon E. "AIDS in Africa: Death is the Only Certainty," and "Missionaries in Africa are Not Immune to AIDS," *Christianity Today*, Vol.32, No.6 (April 8, 1988), pp. 36–40.

24. Preciado, Consuelo. "AIDS and the Five Year Information Gap," *Americas 2001*, Vol 1, no.5 (March/April), 1988, pp.8–17.

25. SAC (Spiritual Advisory Committee). "AIDS: A Spiritual Perspective," from *AIDS: A Self-Care Manual, AIDS Project Los Angeles*, 1987, pp. 215–235.

26. Seibert, Gary. "A Plague, Not a War: The Religious Press Confronts Itself Through AIDS," *America*, Oct.24, 1987.

27. Schaper, Richard L. "Pastoral Care for Persons with AIDS and for their Families," *The Christian Century*, (August 12–19, 1987), pp. 691–694.

28. Stephens, Robert. "Religious Press Urged: Tell the Human Story of AIDS," *Catholic Health World*, Oct. 15, 1987. p. 9.

29. Syme, Leonard S. and Lisa F. Berkman. "Social Class, Susceptibility and Sickness," *American Journal of Epidemiology*, Vol 164, No.1 (1978), pp 1–6.

30. *UC Clip Sheet* (Special issue on AIDS research in the University of California system), vol. 63, no. 20 (UC Berkeley:May,1988).

31. USCC (United States Catholic Conference). "The Many Faces of AIDS: A Gospel Response," (a statement of the Administrative Board of the Conference), Washington, D.C., Nov. 1987.
32. Wood, William. "Teach the Children Well," *America,* May 16,1987.
33. Worth, Dooley and Ruth Rodriguez. "Latina Women and AIDS," *SIECAS Report,* January–February, 1987, pp.5–7.

Personal Interviews

1. Barrett, Father Edward. Roman Catholic Chaplain, Veterans Administration Hospital, West Los Angeles.
2. Bendaña, Lily. Director of educational program for Hispanics commissioned by the Centers for Disease Control, Sosa and Associates, San Antonio, Texas.
3. Benschoter, Ron. Associate Director of Development, AIDS Action Council, Washington, D.C.
4. Bosco, Most Reverend Anthony G., D.D., J.C.L. Member of the National Conference of Catholic Bishops/U.S. Catholic Conference AIDS Task Force and Third Bishop of Greensburg, Pa., Pennsylvania.
5. Caruso, Father Lawrence. Associate Superintendent of Catholic Schools throughout the Los Angeles Archdiocese.
6. Cassidy, Monseignor James Patrick. Director of Health and Hospitals for the Archdiocese of New York and Chancellor of the New York Medical College, New York City.
7. Dalton, Harlon. Professor, Yale Law School, and author, *AIDS and the Law,* New Haven, Ct.
8. Diaz, Eunice. Director of Community Affairs, White Memorial Center, Los Angeles.
9. Gallagher, Father Thomas. United States Catholic Conference Secretary for Education, Washington, D.C.
10. Escobar, Zoila. Health Educator formerly in charge of working with Latino Community, Aids Project Los Angeles.
11. Gigrich, Father John. Associate Pastor at St. Matthew's Cathedral, Coordinator of Pastoral Care of Persons Suffering with AIDS, and Special Assistant to the Archbishop for Ministering to Homosexual Catholics, Washington, D.C.
12. Harris, Sister Jeanne, O.P. Media Utilization Specialist for Telecommunications Services, Los Angeles Archdiocese, Los Angeles.
13. Hughes, Dr. Patrick. Director of Pastoral Ministry for the Archdiocese of San Francisco.
14. Kane, Father Francis. Director of Community Services, Archdioceses of Chicago.
15. Liuzzi, Father Peter. Director of Religious Formation, Carmel West Seminary, Los Angeles.
16. McDermott, Peter. Executive Director of the Serra Ancillary Care Corporation (Los Angeles Archdiocese), Los Angeles.
17. Morrow-Hall, Gavin. Community worker, Minority AIDS Project, Los Angeles.
18. Ochoa, Auxiliary Bishop Armando. Bishop of San Fernando, Los Angeles Archdiocese.
19. O'Connor, Father Matt. Dominican from the Southern Province, St. Ambros Parish, Los Angeles.

20. Power, Sister Jane Francis. Director of Department of Health Affairs, Los Angeles Archdiocese, Los Angeles.
21. Puente, Michael. Assistant Director of AIDS program, Cara A Cara, Los Angeles.
22. Reinhart-Marean, Reverend Tom. Aids Project Los Angeles, Los Angeles.
23. Reyes, Jennie. Eucharistic Minister, Founder of Mothers of People with AIDS, Public Speaker and only Latino board member of the newly formed, Washington-based National AIDS Interfaith Council association, Montebello, CA.
24. Salinas, Raquel. Health Educator, El Centro-Milagro AIDS Project, Los Angeles.
25. Tesconi, Louis. Founder and Director of Damien Ministries, Washington, D.C.
26. Vega, Rafael. President of Dignity, Los Angeles.
27. Zelewsky, Marianne. Coordinator of the AIDS ministry for the Archdiocese of Chicago and community health nurse at Loyola University, Chicago.

Chapter 6

How to Cover a Plague

James Kinsella

FOR MORE THAN TWO YEARS, until mid-1983, the American media largely ignored one of the biggest stories of this century: AIDS. And not until mid-1985, following the death of Rock Hudson, did the epidemic become an item newsworthy enough to become a regular assignment at major newspapers, magazines, and the networks.

Why did almost every journalist overlook this story in the beginning? And why has AIDS come to be covered in the way it has? The answer lies in probably the most basic tenet of decision making in the news business: the closer news moves to affecting news producers or those individuals they perceive as their audience, the greater the news value of the story.

A chart showing the number of AIDS stories produced by a select group of representative media outlets during the early years of the epidemic indicates that coverage leaped during three specific time periods, and dropped off somewhat after each: in mid-1983, mid-1985, and early 1987.[1]

In mid-1983, a study indicating that AIDS may be passed by casual contact, coupled with news about contaminated blood transfusions and children getting the disease, pushed many journalists who had never written about the epidemic to file their first stories. In mid-1985, the publication of Rock Hudson's AIDS diagnosis, an event that seemed to suggest anyone could get the disease, sent the media into paroxysms. And in early 1987, when the mosquito-theory of transmission burst forth, reporters once again pushed the amount of AIDS coverage to an unprecedented level.

What all these stories have in common is that they suggest in some way that AIDS is threatening to spread into the population of White, non-I.V.-drug-using, middle-class Americans, which is the profile of the average journalist and media gatekeeper.

A Note on Methodology

In doing the research for this chapter, and my forthcoming book, I have relied on basic journalistic method. That is, the great majority of my information comes from interviews with people involved in reporting or editing the news. I also have spoken with doctors, scientists, and some government officials who are or were often in news about the AIDS epidemic. My interviews lasted from thirty minutes to eight hours, and almost all of them were done in person.

My assistant and I have closely studied a wide range of news material on the epidemic, from network coverage to the *New York Times'* reporting; from the work of the *New York Native*, a publication for the Gay community, to *Newsweek, Time,* and *U.S. News and World Report.*

Where necessary, I have used research produced by media experts, such as the graph mentioned above that was put together by Don Berreth of the Centers for Disease Control. I indicate with a footnote those instances in which I borrowed information.

The stories that I craft adhere strictly to the facts. Although I avoid the heavy use of quotations, the descriptions and thoughts attributed to certain journalists, doctors, or others come directly from my interviews with them.

Underplaying an Epidemic

In the beginning, when AIDS was considered an exclusively Gay plague, few gatekeepers — indeed, few journalists — felt personally touched by the disease. Thus, they considered the emerging epidemic as something of little interest to their average readers. The next group to be affected, illicit intravenous-drug users, hardly broadened the appeal of the story.

Homophobia and social intolerance were clearly at play at newspapers, magazines, and the networks. In recent interviews, scores of editors have admitted their own uneasiness when dealing with the issue of homosexuality, and that discomfort certainly had an effect on how much coverage Gays, or issues related to that community, could garner.

But even some in the Gay press were reluctant to write about AIDS at first, fearing that any publicity of what might be construed as a negative aspect of the Gay community could result in a backlash from right-wing extremist groups. Hard-won civil rights seemed to hang in the balance. But for the most part, the hesitation among Gay publications to tackle the AIDS issue was temporary. More common among these papers and magazines has been an intense interest. The *New York Native,* for instance, was the first of any American media outlet to run a story on the AIDS crisis.[2]

Still, when reporters from the major print and broadcast outlets share their horror stories about the early years of the epidemic, the tales are rarely about death and dying. Instead, the journalists talk about colleagues whose editors claimed there wasn't room in the paper for news about Gays. Or they remember a TV reporter whose camera crew—

fearing infection — cut the microphone hook-up after she finished interviewing a family caring for an AIDS patient.[3]

But other obstacles served to block adequate coverage of the epidemic. For instance, the story was first and foremost a "science" topic — and few media outlets have journalists on staff who are specifically trained to cover the complex beats of science and medicine. What's more, scientists and doctors often believe it isn't in their best interest to talk to journalists about their groundbreaking work, since researchers want their papers to be published first in scientific journals that can place a professional imprimatur on their findings. Such a stamp of approval from colleagues is often essential for career advancement, and publications like the *New England Journal of Medicine* will reject work that already has been written about extensively in the mainstream media. TV posed another set of problems: AIDS often makes for paltry "visuals." Withering patients are often the only appropriate graphics, and many AIDS victims refuse to appear on camera.

Getting the Story

Homophobia, lack of science expertise, poor reporter-researcher communication, and even inadequate visuals all conspire to keep the AIDS story from being reported as the major breaking news it was. As a result, where and when AIDS was covered in the early years was almost always a result of a reporter's individual initiative. And the connection a particular journalist had with the epidemic became a much stronger influence on what appeared in the news and on what Americans knew about the crisis than was the case with almost any other recent major news story.

On the Frontline

Vincent Coppola had finally gotten his parents to visit Atlanta, where he and his wife and child lived, and where he worked for *Newsweek's* Southeast bureau. His parents were working class people who raised four sons in a cramped Brooklyn home. They were a close family, as families go.

So it wasn't surprising when, during the visit, Vincent's younger brother Thomas called from New York to tell him and his parents he was sick. "I have this thing affecting Haitians, drug addicts . . . and homosexuals," he said.

Coppola hadn't known his brother was Gay. Indeed, he would come to realize he hardly knew his brother at all, before Thomas got sick. That was late 1982. Thomas was twenty-eight years old, a tall husky blond model struggling to become an actor.

Coppola, thirty-four at the time, had been working for *Newsweek* since 1978. He was considered an aggressive and bright reporter who could stretch enough to handle general assignment work. AIDS would become the assignment of his life.

Shortly after Vince hung up the phone on that summer night, he headed for the reference books. He looked up immune deficiency and Kaposi's Sarcoma, the telltale brown spots that the doctors had found on Thomas' feet. Coppola had never heard of a disease that could kill a healthy young man in his prime, and he decided he would help save his brother's life.

In the next few days Coppola read everything he could about Gay-related infectious disease. When he finished that he went to the Centers for Disease Control itself. It was a steamy Georgia day when he marched in, without an appointment, to the office of Dr. James Curran, the man in charge of the nascent AIDS Task Force. Coppola's *Newsweek* connection helped him get past Curran's secretary. It would tumble many more obstacles in the future as Coppola scrambled to learn of the latest research and to get Thomas into the best treatment programs available.

What he was uncovering he was also attempting to get into the pages of *Newsweek* itself. The magazine had done a smattering of stories since late 1981, when it looked into the spread of "Diseases That Plague Gays." But the epidemic didn't gain serious consideration at the magazine until Coppola wrote his first memo about the subject. Indeed, editors and writers involved in reporting the AIDS story at *Newsweek* in the first few years credit that memo for spurring the April 18, 1983 cover, "The AIDS Epidemic: The Search for a Cure." It was the first major treatment of the issue by a national, general interest magazine.

In American journalism, a *Newsweek* cover story does not necessarily set the national agenda for news. The wire services, the *New York Times* and, to a lesser extent, the *Washington Post,* government agencies, even the networks and *USA Today* are cited more frequently by media players as powerful agenda-setting institutions.

But *Newsweek's* impact on the AIDS story in 1983 was significant. *Time* magazine, for instance, quickly followed up with its own cover in July of 1983. The feature treatment the two national newsweeklies gave the epidemic helped to open up a new avenue of reporting on the crisis. It's almost impossible to pinpoint just what kind of interest those two cover stories generated among newspaper and broadcast journalists, but they clearly helped move the story from the science beat and expand the audience for AIDS news.

What if a reporter at the *New York Times,* a journalist for Associated Press, or a correspondent at one of the three major networks had tackled the story aggressively in the summer or fall of 1981? Stories beyond the scientific oddity of a new disease — for example, news about how fear of the unknown was spreading through the Gay communities of big cities — probably would have prompted more reporting on other aspects of the epidemic, including funding for research and necessary preventive actions. "We are all good leeches," a prominent TV executive recently said of the tendency for journalists to follow each other's leads.[4]

That broad approach to reporting happened almost instantaneously when the Centers for Disease Control identified Legionnaire's Disease, a sickness that affected middle-aged war veterans. Of course, the nature of the Legionnaire's outbreak differed substantially from AIDS: it occurred predominantly in one location — a Philadelphia hotel — and the scientific mystery was much easier to solve. Nonetheless, media institutions weren't facing a lack of connectedness to those suffering during that tragedy, as they did in the AIDS epidemic.

Touched by Death

Coppola's connection to the AIDS story was extraordinary, but certainly not unique. Thousands of journalists across the country were also being touched by the plague. After all, many are Gay, or have brothers or friends who were dying from the disease. But Coppola was one of the few willing to act on that connection. Another was Laurie Garrett. When one of her friends came down with the disease in 1983, the National Public Radio correspondent took a new interest in the AIDS story, which showed in the amount and kinds of coverage she was doing. A trained immunologist, she branched out from the science angle to ask questions such as, "Is AIDS research being funded at an adequate level?" Later she would travel to Africa to cover the story in the Third World. And she would return to the U.S. to investigate how AIDS was devastating Third World America.[*] Indeed, Garret was willing to let herself be affected by the death of her friend and the withering of a small child she met in Africa and the despair of a mother from Newark who was watching her family die one by one from the disease.

The Politicized Reporter

Connections like Coppola and Garrett had to the story, and their willingness to act on them, produced some of the best coverage of the plague in America. But there are clear dangers in a reporter being drawn too far into the heart of the story.

Garrett consistently walks a careful line between bloodless journalism and misleading subjectivity. Coppola, devoted to saving his brother, stumbled off that line on occasion. Indeed, his use of his journalist's credentials to smooth the way for his brother seemed at once both understandable and unethical.

Similarly, the reporting by the *San Francisco Chronicle's* Randy Shilts often veered off into less-than-objective territory. Shilts is a Gay man aligned with a political faction in San Francisco's homosexual community, and he reported on the disease and efforts to staunch it in ways that reflected that affiliation.

The Harvey Milk Democratic Club had been named for the San Francisco supervisor murdered by a heterosexual political rival, and the organization was dedicated to promoting the martyr's vision of pragmatic politics. During the first years of the epidemic, those politics seemed to dictate restrictions on the city's Gay bathhouses — where casual, dangerous sex was rampant.

Shilts had grown close to the leaders of the group while he worked on a book detailing Milk's life and rise to influence. Now, as he reported on efforts to rein in the bathhouses, some critics claimed his biases were beginning to show. Indeed, many of Shilts' articles, and some of his actions outside of the *Chronicle*, indicate his support for the Milk Club's agenda. Additionally, Shilt's coverage of the bathhouse debate sometimes appears to have been excessive; it certainly helped make the issue one of the dominant political focuses of 1984 and 1985.

But Shilts and the *Chronicle* undoubtedly helped educate San Franciscans about AIDS. Surveys from mid-1983 to 1987 show significant shifts in the sexual habits of the city's homosexuals.[5] Would a less politicized Shilts have been better for San Francisco? Undeniably, he would have drawn less attention away from the real issues of providing adequate education as well as treatment and long-term care for AIDS patients.

The Freedom to Be a Reporter

Despite the excesses of Randy Shilts, or the clear bias of Vincent Coppola, they produced cutting-edge reporting. They, of course, can't take sole credit. Not only did

---

[*] This term refers to poverty pockets of the United States, such as Newark, New Jersey, or Watts, Los Angeles, which somehow have not been touched by development.

these reporters, and Garrett and a handful of other journalists across the country, have a significant connection to the story and were willing to act on it, but they also had the freedom to do so at their respective media institutions.

A correspondent with less of a reputation than Coppola, or a reporter without mandate to cover the Gay community as Shilts had at the *Chronicle,* or a journalist without the awards Garrett had won for her groundbreaking reporting, would not likely have been able to cover the disease with the depth and breadth these three individuals did.

Getting the Facts Straight

A commitment to the AIDS story did more than produce a quantity of coverage; often it raised the quality, as well. Jim Bunn of KPIX-TV in San Francisco is a good example. He was a general assignment reporter almost completely untrained in science journalism when he began covering the epidemic in 1983.

Yet struck by the growing number of deaths in San Francisco, he and his colleagues took on the AIDS story and produced some of the most accurate AIDS reporting in the broadcast medium. They eventually created the nationally syndicated "AIDS Lifeline," a Peabody Award-winning series of stories and brochures to publicize the threat of AIDS. Indeed, rarely did KPIX make the kind of faux pas common on the networks. For example, in a 1983 broadcast, Peter Jennings mentioned a plant fungus found in the blood of three AIDS victims that seemed to lower the body's resistance to the disease. "Doctors say their research is very preliminary but say they are very excited about it." There was no word on who the doctors were or even whether their study—a study of three people?—was valid. Most egregious of all, there was no follow-up in the days after.

Dan Rather participated in a similar gaffe. A correspondent reported a recall of a blood product for hemophiliacs that was thought to be contaminated with the AIDS virus, but he never specified just what blood product was potentially contaminated. Rather followed up the story the next night, clarifying that the blood product of one specific company was not the dangerous serum. But he never got around to saying just which blood product was in question.[7]

How to Cover a Plague

Detailing these successes and failures is not meant to suggest that any media outlet had a perfect—or perfectly awful—record of covering AIDS. The fact is, almost every major American media has made mistakes, and also has become committed to following the epidemic. As a result, the sophistication of AIDS reporting has improved significantly. The *New York Times* is probably the most dramatic example. For the first two years of the crisis the national paper of record more or less ignored the epidemic, except for an occasional science story by Dr. Lawrence Altman; in the last five years the *Times* has become a showcase for first-rate and extensive AIDS coverage among daily newspapers in the U.S.

Overall, American media has become much less modest about language, a direct result of having to cover a disease that's transmitted largely through sex. In the first few AIDS years, many media outlets hesitated to use "Gay" as a noun. There was also blushing resistance to talking about anal and oral sex. Unfortunately, many doctors and public health officials provided all too convenient – and confusing – terms to allow journalists to write around potentially problematic language. "Exchange of bodily fluids" was one such phrase. But just what does it mean? Appropriate words such as semen, ejaculation, penis, and vagina are increasingly being used to discuss transmission and risk in straightforward ways.

The change in language, of course, was necessary to accommodate new topics. Seven years after the epidemic was first publicized, American media addresses sexual issues in a much more sophisticated manner. Even sociological phenomena like the Gay Rights movement and Gay communities get a broader and more sensitized airing than they did only a half decade ago. There have been dire predictions by pundits like the *New York Times'* Frank Rich, who claimed in *Esquire* recently that AIDS would end the move toward equal rights for Gays. But activists across the country say that the increased media attention – indeed, the sympathy much AIDS coverage has generated – is actually de-stigmatizing Gays.

Journalists and their audiences have learned a great deal from the epidemic. Probably the best way to judge how far the American media has come is to analyze how it would react in 1988 to a story with hysteria-spreading potential like the 1983 study on casual contact. The report by Dr. William Masters and Virginia Johnson, claiming the AIDS virus is far more widespread among non-I.V. drug-using heterosexuals than the government admits, seems well suited for the purpose. Geared more toward advancing royalties than understanding of the epidemic, the book is based on a poorly conducted study and a biased sampling. Indeed, it also grabbed an ideal forum for gaining the attention of journalists: the cover of *Newsweek,* on March 14, 1988. (And it sullied that magazine's good reputation for AIDS coverage in the process.)

But almost no reporter took the bait. In fact, what filled the papers and airwaves was some of the most balanced, and cautious, reporting yet. It was the clear iteration of facts – which is, after all, the most important task of journalists – that proved the best device to put the sexologists' work in perspective.

The Future of the AIDS Beat

Journalists covering AIDS are facing new challenges as the U.S. experiences the epidemic's second wave, in which AIDS is affecting primarily Blacks and Hispanics from America's Third World. In New York City alone there are an estimated 200,000 I.V. drug users, half of them already infected with the virus. When they fall ill – and some researchers strongly believe almost all of them will – they will account for a 200 percent increase in the total AIDS cases throughout the nation.

But coverage of this second wave isn't likely to come easy. Gays in many major metropolitan areas are politically organized and vocal, as well as middle class, White, and literate. In short, they made good, readable copy. The Blacks and Hispanics being infected are often poor, I.V. drug users who pass the disease on to their sexual partners and offspring. And most often these individuals are powerless. If the media is to stay on top of this story, it will have to reach into the communities where the AIDS news is happening: Black ghettos and Hispanic barrios.

The media institution itself will have to change to accommodate a broader diversity of techniques in disseminating information. The reporter is only one conduit; pundits on the editorial page, for example, should recognize their responsibility to educate readers, not only on the political and moral issues of the day but also on the health realities that increasingly will face communities. What's more, "family" papers and broadcast outlets will have to continue to grapple with language issues.

There will come a time when the epidemic is old news. After all, heart disease each year kills many more times the number of Americans killed by AIDS. But there are plenty of stories still to be written, including the use and misuse of AIDS as a campaign issue, the process by which treatments are OK'd or held up, and the threat to the health infrastructure that the disease poses.

None of the above recommendations for the media requires a radical departure from the current mission of many broadcast and print outlets to provide news in the public interest. The suggestions, however, do necessitate that publishers, owners, editors, and reporters take another look at just how they are fulfilling that mandate.

Footnotes

1. The count was done by Don Berreth of the Centers for Disease Control in the spring of 1988, using the Nexis database.
2. "Disease Rumors Largely Unfounded." Dr. Larry Mass. *New York Native.* May 18, 1981.
3. The TV-reporter anecdote was taken from "Editors, Cameramen Make AIDS Reporting Harder Than Necessary," by Laurie Garrett in *The Newsletter of the National Association of Science Writers.* September 1987.
4. In an interview with Bill Lord, executive producer for ABC World News Tonight. April 26, 1988.
5. Several published and unpublished studies indicate this change: "Designing an Effective AIDS Prevention Campaign Strategy: Results from the first and second probability sample of an urban Gay male community," Dec. 3, 1984 and June 28, 1985, San Francisco AIDS Foundation; "Reported Changes in Sexual Behavior of Men at Risk for AIDS," in *Public Health Reporters,* 100, 6, 622, 628, Leon McKusick et al.
6. Oct. 26, 1983, ABC World News Tonight.
7. Aug. 30, 1983, The CBS Evening News, Terry Drinkwarter reporting; Aug. 31, 1983, Dan Rather.

Chapter 7

An Attributional Analysis of Changing Reactions to Persons with AIDS

Bernard Weiner

IT IS QUITE APPARENT that emotional and behavioral reactions to individuals with AIDS are often complex and conflicted, determined by a multiplicity of factors. In this chapter, an analysis of these attitudes is presented, focusing on the historical changes that have transpired and are still occurring in responses toward persons with this affliction. The interpretation that is offered uses principles from attribution theory, a conception based on phenomenal causality, or "why" a particular outcome has come about. Because attribution theory has been a dominant approach within social psychology, it is possible to bring a wealth of empirical evidence and a well-developed set of theoretical tools to the present examination of AIDS.

Causality, Emotion and Action

Attributional analyses begin with an outcome, such as success or failure at an achievement-related task, or social acceptance or rejection. Search is then undertaken to determine the cause of that outcome (see review in Weiner, 1986). Perceived causality, in turn, gives rise to a variety of affects, and also influences the expectancy of goal attainment. Affect and expectancy then play essential roles in determining subsequent behavior. For example, a student may succeed at an exam and ascribe that success to high ability. High ability perceptions elicit pride in accomplishment as well as a high expectancy of future success. Furthermore, student pride, accompanied by a high expectancy of success, generates continued achievement strivings (see review in Weiner, 1986). These processes have been documented not only in self perception, but also in the perception of others. For example, the failure of a pupil may be perceived by a teacher as due to low aptitude. Limited aptitude evokes pity as well as a low expectancy of pupil success. These reactions could then result in the teacher providing concerned counseling, encouraging this student to change career goals. In sum, the general conceptual framework for approaching issues from an attributional perspective is the following:

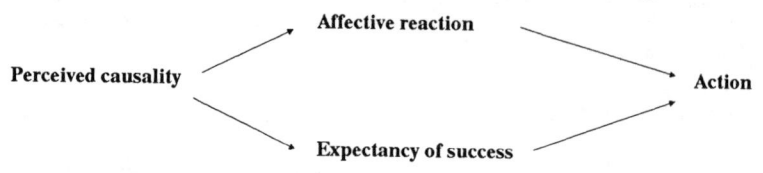

```
                        Affective reaction
                       ↗                  ↘
   Perceived causality                       Action
                       ↘                  ↗
                       Expectancy of success
```

Associations between attributions for the actions of others, affect, expectancy, and behavior also have been documented outside of the achievement domain. One area of particular relevance to attribution theorists has been altruism and the decision to help others (see Schmidt & Weiner, forthcoming). I will soon discuss such prosocial behavior, for it is central to the concerns addressed in this chapter.

Attributional Theory Applied to AIDS

Reactions to individuals with AIDS, the topic of this chapter, also are amenable to the attributional analysis suggested above; i.e., an interpretation that includes perceived causality, affective responses, expectancies about the future, and intended or actual action. For an attributional analysis to be applicable, the assumption first must be imposed that AIDS, which is a social stigma, itself represents a negative outcome. Given the recognized adverse consequences of AIDS, such an assumption is quite reasonable.

Much research has revealed that negative outcomes or effects, such as achievement failure or social rejection, particularly initiate attributional search (see review in Weiner, 1986). Considering social stigmas such as AIDS, search is presumed to be undertaken by the stigmatized person as well as by others (observers) to determine the origin of the disease. Thus, people with AIDS frequently ask themselves the existential attribution, "Why me?" while others may search for a more immediate and direct causal explanation. But for AIDS, the disease itself implies a cause and is associated with an attribution, thus negating the need for further search. The cause most likely to be brought to mind is broadly conceived as "moral weakness," and more specifically is homosexual behavior and/or drug use. According to attribution theory, the perceived causes of AIDS should (and do!) then determine affective reactions toward that person (e.g., pity and anger), future expectancies regarding the individual (e.g., the likelihood of recovery), and a variety of behavioral responses including, for example, charity donations and personal assistance. Let us therefore explore in greater detail what these reactions might be, and how they relate to help-giving and prosocial behavior.

Attributions and Help-Giving

The relationship between attributions, emotions, and action has been extensively investigated with regard to help-giving. For example, in a series of help-related investigations, an individual was described to a research subject as having fallen in a subway. In one of the manipulated conditions of the study, the person in need of aid was characterized as drunk, while in a second condition the needy person was portrayed as ill. Respondents indicated that they would feel disgust and anger toward the drunk person, in addition to experiencing a small amount of pity. Further, they stated that they would tend not to offer help. On the other hand, respondents indicated that in the case of an ill person they would have a great deal of sympathy, little anger, and would extend help. In a similar series of hypothetical vignettes, a student was described as asking to borrow class notes of the respondent. In one of the experimental conditions, the student hadn't taken the notes because he "went to the beach," while in a second condition the notes were not taken because the student had eye problems. The college participants indicated that their responses to the "beach" student would be anger, little sympathy, and neglect, while reactions to the student with eye problems would be sympathy, help-giving, and no anger; (these and other pertinent investigations are reviewed in Weiner, 1986).

In the two series of studies briefly summarized above, reports of anger, sympathy (pity), and helping were mediated by perceptions regarding the cause of a need. The essential difference between these two experimental conditions concerns perceived responsibility for the onset of the need. The lazy student and the drunk on the subway were both held responsible (able to respond) for their plights, while the ill person and the student with eye problems were not personally blamed for their negative states. This property of causality has been labeled "controllability," and connotes whether the cause of a state such as falling or lack of notes is perceived as subject to personal command or volitional alteration. Based on the sketched investigations, two behavioral sequences relating perceptions of controllability to emotional reactions and behavior have been documented:

1. Controllable need ⟶ anger toward the other ⟶ neglect

2. Uncontrollable need ⟶ sympathy toward the other ⟶ neglect

Of course, help-related behavior and pertinent affective reactions are also influenced by factors other than perceived causality. One might fear the drunk, there may be social norms to help all other students, there could be perceived personal costs and benefits from helping others, and so on. In this chapter I will refer to the myriad of these variables as *nonattributional* determinants of emotion and action. These nonattributional determinants could augment or decrease emotional responding and help-giving. With these principles in mind, I now will consider the feelings and behaviors that have been directed toward those with AIDS. I will be especially concerned with historical changes in these reactions and how they are mediated by changes in attributional determinants — perceptions regarding causality.

Reactions to AIDS Considered from an Attributional Perspective

When AIDS was initially reported in 1981, relatively little organized intervention was undertaken. The slow acknowledgment of this disease has been the subject of much criticism directed at the United States and other governments. Clearly, one reason for the inaction was that little was known or appreciated about the illness. Even after some initial understanding was reached, however, there was still limited responsivity. Guided by the perspective presented above, it is argued that AIDS was ignored because of both attribution-mediated and nonattributional determinants. The attribution-related determinant was that AIDS was perceived as onset-controllable; the persons contracting this illness were held personally responsible and blamed. Hence, individuals in this state elicited anger, relatively little pity, and neglect from others. The nonattributional determinant of neglect, which will not be further examined in this context, was the association of this disease with homosexuality (and shortly thereafter with drug use). Independent of the perceived controllability of these actions, the behaviors per se are not condoned in our society and elicit negative reactions. This initial stage in the historical analysis of reactions to AIDS is shown in Table 1.

Table 1. HISTORICAL ANALYSIS OF REACTIONS TO PERSONS WITH AIDS

Stage 1 (1981–1984):
[a] AIDS — onset controllable — little pity, some anger — neglect
[b] AIDS — contracted by gay males — sexual hostility — little pity, anger — neglect

Stage 2 (1985):
[a] AIDS — onset controllable — little pity, some anger — neglect
[b] AIDS — contracted by gay males — sexual hostility — little pity, anger — neglect
[b] AIDS — perceptions of communicability — anger — aggression

Stage 3 (1985–1987):
[a] AIDS — onset controllable — little pity, some anger — neglect
[b] AIDS — contracted by gay males — sexual hostility — little pity, anger — neglect
[b] AIDS — perceptions of communicability — anger — aggression
[b] AIDS — perceptions of communicability — fear — nonaltruistic help

Stage 4 (1987–present):
[a] AIDS — onset controllable — little pity, some anger — neglect
[b] AIDS — contracted by gay males — sexual hostility — little pity, anger — neglect
[b] AIDS — perceptions of communicability — anger — aggression
[b] AIDS — perceptions of communicability — fear — nonaltruistic help
[a] AIDS — onset uncontrollability — pity, no anger — altruistic help

[a] Attributionally - mediated reactions
[b] Nonattributionally - mediated reactions

In a recent series of experiments using both American subjects and Canadian residents, we presented the participants with ten stigmas to consider, including AIDS. We asked our respondents the perceived controllability of this stigma and how much they would blame the stigmatized person, the amount of anger and pity they would experience toward these individuals, and whether they would personally help or be charitable toward them. These data are shown in Table 2. Table 2 reveals that AIDS is perceived as onset-controllable; that is, the person with this illness is perceived as responsible and blamed. Thus, AIDS is classified with stigmas such as obesity and child abuse, rather than with Alzheimer's disease, blindness, cancer, and the like. Furthermore, individuals with AIDS elicit rather little liking and pity, some anger, and relatively little personal assistance and charitable donations. Note, however, that persons with AIDS do elicit more pity and indications of charity than persons with other stigmas that are perceived as controllable. I believe this is due to the terminal nature of this illness, as well as the fact that AIDS is perceived as having a controllable onset but an uncontrollable offset.

Table 2. MEAN VALUES FOR TEN STIGMAS

Stigma	\multicolumn{7}{c}{Controllability-Related Variables}
	Responsibility	Blame	Like	Pity	Anger	Assistance	Charit Donations
Alzheimer's	.8^a	.5^a	6.5^{bc}	7.9^a	1.4^e	8.0^a	6.9^{bc}
Blind	.9^a	.5^a	7.5^a	7.4^a	1.7^e	8.5^a	7.2^{abc}
Cancer	1.6^{ab}	1.3^{ab}	7.6^a	8.0^a	1.6^e	8.4^a	8.1^a
Heart Disease	2.5^b	1.6^b	7.5^a	7.4^a	1.6^e	8.0^a	7.5^{ab}
Paraplegic	1.6^{ab}	.9^{ab}	7.0^{ab}	7.6^a	1.4^e	8.1^a	7.1^{abc}
Vietnam War Syndrome	1.7^{ab}	1.5^b	5.7^c	7.1^a	2.1^e	7.0^b	6.2^{cd}
AIDS	4.4^c	4.8^c	4.8^d	6.2^b	4.0^c	5.8^c	6.5^{bc}
Child Abuse	5.2^c	6.0^{de}	2.0^f	3.3^d	7.9^a	4.6^d	4.0^f
Drug Abuse	6.5^d	6.7e	3.0^e	4.0^d	6.4^b	5.3^{cd}	5.0^e
Obesity	5.3^c	5.2^{cd}	5.7^c	5.1^c	3.3^d	5.8^c	4.0^f
F Values	96.02*	156.85*	108.60*	59.31*	157.76*	44.88*	42.59*

*$p < .001$
means not sharing any subscript differ at the $p < .01$ level

A short time later, when AIDS began to spread and its communicability—as well as its threat to the heterosexual population—became more evident, anger towards the carriers of this disease began to flourish. As Triplet and Sugarman (1987) summarized:

> ...Homosexual rights legislation that was pending in several state legislatures has been tabled in the face of acrimonious debate...., a Gallop poll has indicated that attitudes towards homosexuals have generally become more negative...,and Haitian immigrants have faced increasing discrimination in housing and employment....Even among college students, a traditionally tolerant segment of the population, 47.8% currently approve of legislation prohibiting homosexual relations (pp. 265-266).

Furthermore, there was an alarming growth of aggressive action that has been directly traced to "retaliation" for the carrying and spreading of AIDS by homosexuals. Thus, not only was AIDS perceived by some as a form of "revenge" from God, but having the disease itself promotes further human reprisal. Paradoxically, the "punishment" itself provoked further punishment! These reactions to AIDS are shown inStage 2 of Table 1.

As personal fear began to grow because of the communicability of this illness, however, private and governmental support soon also was augmented. This is illustrated in the following report from the *New York Times:*

> "In the last six months, there has been an enormous change in the responses of foundations, corporations, and the public generally," said Dr. Mathilde Krim, a research biologist who established the AIDS Medical Foundation in 1983. "I cannot pinpoint any single event or reason, but people finally have caught on that AIDS is a potential threat to everybody and has an impact on health, the economy, and our lives," said Dr. Krim, who has frequently complained about the public apathy toward the spread of the disease (Teltsch, *New York Times,* July 28, 1987, p. 9).

Hence, the help that was provided was not altruistically motivated; it was driven by concerns and fears for the self, rather than for the afflicted individuals. This analysis characterizes the current, or perhaps just-passed, situation, as shown in Stage 3 of Table 1. Note that in Stage 3 of the hypothesized historical sequence, there are two nonattributional determinants of responding (negative attitudes towards homosexuals and perceptions of communicability) and one attributional source related to perceived controllability. Two influences contribute to neglect and one to aggression; only fear of transmission produces help-giving although, as already indicated, this should be considered self-protecting help and not necessarily prosocial behavior in terms of motivational source.

AIDS now continues to be perceived as contracted by Gay males and drug users, and therefore is still considered onset-controllable. At the same time, however, it is being construed as onset-*un*controllable—infecting blood recipients, infants of parents with AIDS, and heterosexuals engaging in "normal" sexual activity. Although even sexually "innocent" victims can be held somewhat responsible, as evidenced by the increasing advertisements for preventive care, heterosexuals are held less responsible for becoming infected with AIDS than are homosexuals (Triplet & Sugarman, 1987).

My colleagues and I (Weiner, Perry, and Magnusson, in press) have conducted a number of studies in which controllable or uncontrollable reasons are supplied for the onset of a stigma, and then have examined how these information manipulations influence judgments of blame, affective reactions of pity and anger, and help-giving judgments. For example, respondents are told either that cancer was due to unknowingly living in a toxic dump area or was caused by excessive smoking, that heart disease was caused by a genetic deficit or poor diet, that obesity was caused by a thyroid problem or excessive eating with little exercise and—most central to the present topic—that AIDS was caused by either a blood transfusion or engaging in homosexual activity. The judgments made by our respondents are given in Table 3. To explain this rather complex table, and now just concentrating on the AIDS data, Table 3 shows that if AIDS is caused by homosexual activity, the person with the illness is held responsible ($\overline{X} = 6.7$) and personally blamed ($\overline{X} = 6.2$). Indeed, this causal information results in greater perceptions of responsibility

An Attributional Analysis of Changing Reactions to Persons With AIDS

and blame than for any other stigma given any onset-controllable information. If AIDS is described as due to a blood transfusion, however, the person is not at all held responsible ($\bar{X} = .60$) or blamed ($\bar{X} = .80$). Inspection of Table 3 indicates that this is the least blame for any stigma given any information. Thus, AIDS is the most labile stigma in terms of responsibility and blame toward the victim. In a similar manner, the reactions of liking, pity, anger, personal assistance, and charity donations all are influenced by the information manipulation. If AIDS is perceived as uncontrollable, then the person is liked, elicits a great deal of pity, little anger, much personal assistance, and a great deal of charity. The reverse holds true when the cause of AIDS is perceived as controllable. Furthermore, given no information and only the stigma label of AIDS, the person tends to be judged as responsible ($\bar{X} = 5.2$) and blamed ($\bar{X} = 5.2$). That is, our information manipulation of homosexual activity is what is usually called forth in the minds of individuals when this disease is perceived.

Table 3. MEAN VALUES FOR TEN STIGMAS ON SEVEN VARIABLES RELATED TO PERCEIVED CONTROLLABILITY

Stigmas	Condition[1]	Resp	Blame	Like	Pity	Anger	Assist	Charit Donat
Alzheimers	c	(3.6[2]	(3.1	5.8	(6.7	2.5	7.3	(5.9
	uc	0.9)	1.1)	5.9	7.5)	2.0	7.7	6.7)
	ni	1.2	1.4	6.3	7.1	2.4	7.3	6.3
Blind	c	(6.6	(6.3	(4.4	(4.9	(3.9	(6.5	(4.8
	uc	1.1)	0.8)	6.5)	7.6)	1.6)	7.9)	6.8)
	ni	1.5	1.3	6.9	6.7	1.9	7.9	6.7
Cancer	c	6.1	5.0	(4.9	(5.3	(4.0	(6.3	(5.3
	uc	(1.2)	(1.3)	6.2)	7.5)	1.8)	7.5)	7.0)
	ni	2.7	2.6	6.9	6.9	2.2	7.5	6.9
Heart Disease	c	(6.5	(5.0	(4.7	(4.7	(3.8	(5.9	(4.4
	uc	1.0)	1.0)	6.4)	7.0)	1.6)	7.4)	6.3)
	ni	3.4	2.9	6.6	6.3	2.1	7.3	6.1
Paraplegic	c	(5.9	(5.2	(5.1	(5.9	(3.9	(6.8	(5.2
	uc	0.7)	0.9)	6.3)	7.4)	1.6)	7.6)	6.6)
	ni	2.1	2.3	6.4	7.1	2.0	7.7	6.7
Vietnam War Syndrome	c	(3.1	(2.7	(5.2	6.5	2.6	6.9	(5.5
	uc	1.8)	1.7)	5.8)	7.0	2.3	7.2	6.4)
	ni	1.2	1.6	6.2	6.8	2.2	7.4	6.5
AIDS	c	(6.7	(6.2	(3.5	(4.9	(4.2	(4.8	(4.2
	uc	0.6)	0.8)	5.9)	8.2)	1.8)	7.1)	6.9)
	ni	5.2	5.2	4.8	6.0	3.6	5.2	5.5
Child Abuse	c	6.5	6.4	2.4	(3.8	7.2	4.4	2.8
	uc	(5.6)	(5.6)	3.0	5.0)	6.7	4.9	(3.1)
	ni	5.4	5.2	2.9	4.4	6.7	4.9	3.7
Drug Abuse	c	6.4	6.2	3.7	(4.5	(4.7	5.4	3.6
	uc	4.1	4.1	4.8	5.5)	3.1)	6.2	4.2
	ni	6.4	6.1	4.0	4.7	5.2	4.9	4.0
Obesity	c	(6.4	(5.9	(4.6	(4.6	(3.3	5.8	(3.2
	uc	2.6)	2.5)	5.4)	6.3)	2.4)	6.6	4.7)
	ni	5.2	4.8	5.9	5.5	2.7	6.3	4.0

[1] c = controllable information; uc = uncontrollable information; ni = no information.
[2] Couplings indicate a significant difference between conditions ($p < .01$).

It is evident from Table 3 that the perception of AIDS as uncontrollable does increase prosocial responses towards individuals with this illness. Hence, because of the present increase in uncontrollable AIDS, there theoretically also should be an increase in attributionally-mediated reactions of pity and help towards those with this illness (Stage 4, Table 1). That is, help should not only be extended because of personal fear, as in Stage 3. Most helping theorists would consider only Stage 4 as capturing altruistic help because, unlike Stage 3, help is not in service of the help-provider. At the same time, those with onset-controllable AIDS, such as Gay men, still will elicit anger because of their "moral failure," their perceived role as communicators of the disease, and the general negative reactions to homosexuals. It should be noted that in Stage 4 there are two non-attributional sources of public reactions (fear and homophobia) and two attributional sources of reactions (controllable and uncontrollable perceptions).

At the time of this writing, it appears that perceptions of controllability and responsibility are still dominant, although other reactions also are being reported. The August 30, 1987 *New York Times* contained the following survey data:

> The Gallup respondents also were asked to reflect on the responsibility for AIDS. In specific terms, 45 percent agreed that 'most people with AIDS have only themselves to blame,' while 13 percent disagreed. Asked more generally about the cause of the disease, 42 percent agreed with the statement 'I sometimes think that AIDS is a punishment for the decline in moral standards.' Forty-three percent disagreed, saying they did not sometimes hold that view. (Staff, 1987, p. 12).

The Story of the Ray Children

The varied feelings and attitudes described in Stage 4 were recently evidenced in a well-publicized story. Three hemophiliac children contracted AIDS through blood transfusions. Many of the townspeople then did not want these children admitted into the local school. Eventually, after the family house was burned down, the family made a decision to leave and find a more hospitable environment. The *New York Times* (August 31, 1987) reported the following observations, with the concerned article entitled: "To Neighbors of Shunned Family, AIDS Fear Outweighs Sympathy."

> When it was found that the boys had been exposed to AIDS, presumably through the transfusion of blood products they needed to ease the effects of their hemophilia, the School Board barred them from classes[1]... "There isn't anyone who doesn't feel sympathy for the Ray children," said Sue Ellen Smith, the wife of the Mayor of this ranching and citrus community of 6,000. ....Today, the committee formed to close the schoolhouse doors to the three Ray boys who are hemophiliacs, offered donations of food and clothing to the family.

---

[1] The order in the inital paragraph does not correspond to the order in the written article, but has been changed to illustrate the theoretical sequence.

[These statements illustrate the attributional path between uncontrollability, sympathy, and help.]

[Ms. Smith continues] "But there are too many unanswered questions about this disease, and if you are intelligent and listen and read about AIDS you get scared when it involves your own children, because you realize all the assurances are not based on solid evidence." [This traces the path from communicability to fear.]

Today, first inspection had still not determined what caused the fire that razed the Ray house Friday night and convinced the family that Arcadia was no longer their home. Mr. Ray, who said the family had been getting telephone threats, believes it was arson. [This completes the path from communicability to anger and aggression.]

Others were more pointed in their remarks. Herschel, who retired to Arcadia eight years ago from Tennessee, nodded as he talked about the "plague" which he said homosexuals had brought about, adding, "They pass it onto decent people. They should quarantine every one of 'em, isolate them just like they would do with measles or chickenpox." "Yeah, said his partner, anger setting his jaws. They "want" everyone to have some of it. [This apparently illustrates both the non-attributional path from sexual hostility to little pity, anger, and neglect, and from perceived onset controllability when AIDS afflicts homosexuals to anger and neglect]. (Nordheimer, *New York Times,* August 31, 1987, pp. 1, 14).

In sum, while I have taken some liberties in interpretation because of the lack of necessary information, the above story seems to capture both the attributional and nonattributional determinants of the feelings, attitudes, and actions of the individuals towards the Ray children.

The Future

It is quite likely that Stage 4 will soon give way to yet another short-lived stage in the near future, for the perceived nature and course of AIDS is in flux. Some recent evidence suggests that the spread of AIDS among heterosexuals is less than anticipated. Coupled with the new blood detection methods and increasing abortions to potential mothers with AIDS, this could result in a shift back from Stage 4 to Stage 3. That is, AIDS will no longer also be perceived as onset-uncontrollable. This might then have quite negative consequences for help-giving and sources of financial support, inasmuch as altruistic origins of help-giving would be anticipated to stop.

This is rather dramatically revealed in the following report:

> Another federal physician put it more bluntly: "Everybody has got their own agenda, and the thing that fuels the resources for AIDS is the threat of heterosexual transmission. The people who are spending money basically don't care if a bunch of Gay men and drug users get AIDS. They really don't. So the thing that's driving the money is the fear of heterosexual transmission. And the people who run the laboratories that get the money know that. (Scheer, *Los Angeles Times*, Aug. 14, 1987, p. 18).

Conversely, as has been recently argued by Masters and Johnson, perhaps AIDS will rise dramatically among the heterosexual population. Fear as well as perceptions of uncontrollability should then increase, resulting in a great influx of contributions, and demands on the government to take preventive action.

Regardless of the actual future course of events, in all cases the attribution theorist asks: Is the onset of the illness perceived as under volitional control or not? This then determines subsequent affective reactions and help-related behaviors.

References

1. Nordheimer, J. (1987, August 31). "To neighbors of shunned family, AIDS fear outweighs sympathy." *New York Times*, Pt. 1, pps. 1, 14.
2. Scheer, R. (1987, Aug. 14). "AIDS: Is widespread threat an exaggeration?" *Los Angeles Times*, Pt. 1, pp. 1, 18.
3. Schmidt, G., & Weiner, B. (in press). "An attribution-affect action theory of motivated behavior: Replications examining judgments of help-giving." *Personality and Social Psychology Bulletin*.
4. Staff (1987, Aug. 30). "Public is polled on AIDS." *New York Times*, Pt. 1, p. 12.
5. Teltsch, K. (1987, July 28). "Foundations increase support for AIDS patients." *New York Times*, Pt. 1, p. 9.
6. Triplet, R.G., & Sugarman, D.B. (1987). "Reactions to AIDS victims: Ambiguity breeds contempt." *Personality and Social Psychology Bulletin, 13,* 265–274.
7. Weiner, B. (1985). "An attributional theory of achievement motivation and emotion." *Psychological Review, 92,* 548–573.
8. Weiner, B. (1986). *An Attributional Theory of Motivation and Emotion.* New York: Springer-Verlag.
9. Weiner, B., Perry, R., & Magnusson, J. (in press). "An attributional analysis of reactions to stigmas." *Journal of Personality and Social Psychology.*

Chapter 8

Social Consequences of AIDS: Implications for East Africa and the Eastern United States[*]

Francis Paine Conant

ALTHOUGH THE HUMAN IMMUNODEFICIENCY VIRUSES (HIVs) that cause AIDS have spread worldwide and have raised problems of international travel, the granting of visas, and student screening,[1] the social consequences of AIDS and HIV infection are largely evident at much more local levels: for example, a borough in a particular city or, more rarely, a particular countryside within a larger region. In this paper I attempt something new in that I consider the local social consequences of HIV transmission and the frank expression of AIDS in two regions, East Africa and the eastern United States. For present purposes, I include the Atlantic states and make tangential reference to Caribbean and Central American countries.

These regions in two different continents are so different in their environmental, social, and cultural backgrounds that the comparison seems an unlikely one to make, except for this reason: similarities in patterned responses often become evident only when

---

[*] Reprinted from *AIDS 1988: AAAS Symposium Papers,* Ruth Kulstad, ed. (AAAS, Washington, DC, 1988). Reprinted by permission.

considered in alien settings. This holds true also for discovering potential social consequences of HIV infection and AIDS.

The premise here is that the experience of AIDS in one region is now (or soon will be) relevant to the people of another region, even though the two regions may be half a world apart. Their relevance to each other may be in terms of designing educational and other preventive measures to slow HIV transmission or it may be in terms of predicting and perhaps thereby avoiding disruptive political, legal, and social actions. Here I suggest that the effects of AIDS can be looked at in terms of two paradigms: one for the size of the groups affected by a person or persons with HIV infection or AIDS, and the other for coping strategies by individuals or groups, including governments (Table 1).

Table 1. Paradigms for size of groups affected by AIDS and strategies for coping with AIDS

Size of AIDS-Affected Group	Coping Strategies
1. The individual	*Passive:*
2. The couple	A. Acknowledgement
3. Family, household	B. Disavowal, denial
4. Clan	C. Labeling
5. Age groups	*Active:*
6. Occupational class	D. Suppressive
7. Ethnic group	E. Supportive
8. Urban population	F. Scapegoating
9. Rural population	G. Isolating
10. Regional population	H. Quarantine of the afflicted
11. National population	I. Quarantine of the healthy
12. Continental population	*Violent:*
13. Hemispheric population	J. Defiance
	K. Suicide
	L. Group violence
	M. Flight, exodus
	N. Group suicide
	O. Pogrom, genocide

The two paradigms are partly conjectural in the sense that reactions to HIV infection and AIDS have not yet occurred on the scale of the more extreme group sizes and strategies, although they may do so. The paradigms also are differently inflected and scaled so that a position on one does not predict a position on the other. They are suggestive of escalations in size of groups affected by persons with AIDS or HIV infection and in terms of increasingly severe responses. One escalation does not necessarily lead to the next: AIDS in a generation or age group (No. 5) does not inevitably lead to AIDS in an occupational group (No. 6). Similarly, in terms of coping strategies, a consequence of positive support for AIDS patients (E) does not necessarily lead to (F) scapegoating. The "size paradigm" inflects toward increasing inclusiveness; the "coping paradigm" from rather passive strategies to those that are active or violent, or both.

Consideration of the size paradigm is at the level of the individual, the couple, and the family or household; somewhat briefer attention is paid to clan, occupational groups, ethnic groups, and urban and rural populations. Coping strategies are first discussed in the context of the size paradigm and then are given separate consideration with emphasis on labeling, scapegoating, and the more extreme strategies such as isolation, de facto quarantine, and violence.

The Individual

The coping strategies used by the individual in East Africa are affected by at least these three factors: the availability of alternative health care systems, as in recourse to indigenous healers; the economics of public health, which simply do not permit long-term hospitalization of the terminally ill; and the availability of kin or other support groups for assistance to the individual. Similarly, in the eastern United States there is alternative health care in the sense of patients and physicians running their own trials of drugs thought useful in controlling the progress of HIV infection and AIDS, as well as "wild card" treatments bordering on fraud.[2] In the eastern United States AIDS patients are being concentrated in special wards or hospice facilities,[3] but as the number of AIDS patients increases, the next step might well be an East African strategy for the individual: return home to die, or suicide. Anecdotal accounts relate that shame over uncontrollable diarrhea is one reason for suicide by AIDS-affected persons in East Africa. Loneliness and depression are given as causes for suicide or as the basis of claims for the right to die in the eastern United States,[4] but shame and fear of being shamed over change or loss of body functions cannot be ruled out either.

The similarities of some coping strategies between East Africa and the eastern United States are all the more remarkable because of the great difference in transmission modes: in the latter, until recently, transmission was seen as mainly homosexual and via the drug users' contaminated needles. In East Africa, transmission is seen as heterosexual and through contaminated blood supplies used in transfusions. At the outset of the AIDS epidemic in the United States the stigma attached to homosexuality led some individuals to hide or disguise the symptoms of the disease, and this perhaps contributed to official disregard and even denial of the seriousness of the situation. Misguided speculations about a similar origin for AIDS among hypothesized African homosexuals evoked strong reactions by East African governments leading to the same strategy of denial or disavowal of the seriousness of AIDS, and, initially, refusal to cooperate with the World Health Organization. Disavowal strategies in both regions have since moderated toward much more open recognition of AIDS and supportive strategies for resolving AIDS related problems.[5]

The Couple

Coping strategies for couples include scapegoating, isolation, and violence in both eastern Africa and eastern United States regions. As individuals or as couples the differences in power relations between men and women make it likely that women more than men will suffer in the scapegoating process.[6] Men are forgiven for sexual adventures, women are not. Although there has been an official appeal in East Africa for "zero grazing" by men and in the United States for "monogamy" and even abstinence,[7] the double standard still applies. Sexually active men, married or not, are not held responsible for controlling their sexual urges, and are forgiven their adventures. Women are not. They are held responsible not only for their own sexual activities but also for those of their men. In programs aimed at modifying sexual behavior so as to prevent or to slow HIV transmission, women are being targeted as responsible for men's use of condoms. In Hispanic and Black neighborhoods of eastern United States cities there are anecdotal accounts of battering and violence against women who even suggest condom use by their sexual partners.

Scapegoating by labeling is extensive. In the cities of both East Africa and the eastern United States women as prostitutes are seen as central to viral transmission. In the epidemiological literature for East and Central Africa the labels "prostitute," "free woman," or *femme libre* are being used for women who are sexually active outside of a monogamous marriage relationship.[8] The prostitute label is being applied regardless of the multiple, complex roles of women not only in the "barracks" cities of East Africa but also in some cities of the eastern United States. The emergence of these roles in Nairobi has been well studied,[9] and it is evident that continued use of the prostitute label not only distorts the complexity of the social factors involved in HIV transmission but also, because of the pejorative nature of the label, directs attention to women's immorality as a source of HIV transmission rather than the men's sexual adventuring.

In the eastern United States there is a remarkable variation of HIV prevalence among "prostitutes," possibly related to "class" of trade. No workers for an escort service in Miami were HIV positive whereas 41 percent of 90 "inner-city" women prostitutes were.[10] For married women not involved in extramarital sex, there is anecdotal evidence from East Africa that, on discovery of seropositivity or of frank AIDS, such a wife may be faced with abandonment, divorce, or return to her natal kin group. In the eastern United States a wife with AIDS may well find herself in a similar situation, perhaps further complicated by the use of drugs (by herself or by her husband) and, possibly, by his or her bisexual involvements.

The Household, Family, and Clan

At the level of AIDS sickness within the family or household, more active and even violent coping strategies are becoming apparent. In the eastern United States there are accounts of families with AIDS-affected children finding it necessary to move to new communities.[11] Children with AIDS in the eastern United States school system are at the center of legal cases over their presence in the classroom. At least one school with AIDS-affected students has received bomb threats.[12] Very young children with AIDS are sheltered in hospitals because few foster parents or homes will accept them and their adoption is hardly even considered.[13] The extended family in the eastern United States lacks the status it enjoys in East Africa, where the network of kin and links between households can extend from city to countryside and from one remote area to another. It is this network of kin which may provide some shelter for the AIDS-afflicted wife In East Africa.

In eastern United States public ideology, "the family" consists only of monogamously reproducing parents and their children. In East Africa the family may be extended generationally to include grandparents and grandchildren and laterally to include multiple spouses (most commonly a man and more than one woman, but also a woman with more than one man, especially under migrant labor conditions). Large and complex households may join together so that sibling households (linked by brothers and sisters) retain close connections to each other. The potential for helping the household or family member stricken by AIDS seems greater in East African populations than in the eastern United States. The reception in the eastern United States region of someone returning to the natal or home kin group has not been kind,[14] and possibly the same is true in East Africa. The strategies used by these family units in both regions for coping with AIDS need study. They may provide far less costly and perhaps more humane treatment for persons with AIDS than is available in public institutions.

Occupational Group

Some fears have been expressed about AIDS mortality rates "hollowing out" younger African adults in elite government, professional, and commercial occupations. Quite possibly such fears overlook the robustness of the elite cadres in Africa and the capability of the educational system to provide replacements. Similar fears have been expressed in the eastern United States with respect to the entertainment professions and decorative arts. Such concerns perhaps have deflected attention from the effects of AIDS on less prestigious groups such as unskilled laborers (including women) in both the eastern United States and East Africa.[15]

Urban-Rural Populations and Ethnic Groups

AIDS in both the eastern United States and East Africa is known mainly from its expression in urban populations. Despite great differences in cultural origins and relative wealth, there are strong similarities between eastern United States cities and those of East Africa that are likely to affect the consequences of AIDS in both regions. One similarity is that there is uneven distribution of AIDS in residential areas. Men, women, and children in Black and Hispanic sections of eastern United States cities are more affected by AIDS than other groups in other areas of the same city.[16] Equivalent information on East African cities is less clear, but initially one would expect a concentration of cases in the "barracks" or poorer urban areas where social services are few, health conditions are poor, and there are high rates of venereal disease.[17]

Cities of both the eastern United States and East Africa contain populations which maintain relatively intense connections with people in other cities or in rural areas, some of them at great distances from the urban centers. Thus the spread of AIDS from one city to another or from a city to a rural area (and vice versa) seems assured. Rural populations, in fact, may represent something of a stable reservoir of seroprevalence for the AIDS virus [see Nzilambi, *et al.* in reference 8]. In the eastern United States, interurban connections and movement are more intense than urban-rural connections, with the possible exception of migrant farm workers drawn from urban centers. Peoples of the Caribbean basin, including Central America, have intense connections with kin and non-kin in eastern United States cities. Urban-rural, rural-rural, and interurban interconnections are all potential if not actual transmission routes for the spread of the AIDS virus in both East Africa and the eastern United States.

A possibly complicating factor in AIDS virus transmission found in the urban centers of both East Africa and the eastern United States are the large enclaves of expatriates maintaining contact with metropolitan centers on other continents. The United Nations headquarters in New York and the U.N. environmental agencies located in Nairobi are just two cases in point; multinational corporations and their staffs also contribute to the density of intercontinental urban connections. Interurban, intercontinental HIV transmission seems assured[2].

More Active and Some Extreme Coping Strategies

In both the eastern United States and East Africa an initial response to AIDS was denial. In the U.S. region the lack of a vigorous response by federal health agencies has been documented.[18] Pressure from homosexual rights groups, together with the death of several nationally-known performers (Hudson and Liberace), led to public and government acknowledgment of the seriousness of AIDS, together with additional labels referring to it in the print media as a "Gay disease." Prior to this it was the "Haitian disease" or the "Haitian-Black-Drug-Users disease." Labeling in East Africa has followed the same course, but in milder terms: "Slim's disease" refers not only to the loss of weight accompanying AIDS but also to the European expatriate, always concerned with remaining fashionably slim. Apparently everywhere in the East African region the vocabulary referring to AIDS is borrowed, thereby emphasizing its exogenous origin.

Temporary suppression of information about AIDS occurs in both East Africa and the eastern United States until pressure builds to the point of forcing its release. In both regions research in government laboratories must be cleared for publication. The clearing process itself is a way to delay information judged untimely and likely to cause public unrest. There may also be economic reasons for suppressing AIDS information, perhaps from fear of losing revenues from tourism, or the loss of commitments from international agencies and multinational corporations. In the eastern United States there is considerable uneasiness among emergency health and laboratory workers over delays in releasing reports on cases of HIV transmission acquired in the line of duty.[20]

Active and supportive strategies (encouraging AIDS research and proving health and counseling facilities for seropositive persons or those with AIDS) have diverged in East Africa and the eastern United States, as one might expect, according to the differences in public health funds available in the two regions. In the East Africa region supportive measures are limited by public health budgets, and within those budgets a compelling need to counter other, more outstanding threats to health such as malaria and tuberculosis. The East African region is largely dependent on external funding sources for AIDS research and programs to slow transmission of the virus.

The more extreme coping strategies including quarantine (of persons with AIDS or infected with HIV first and, perhaps later, the remaining healthy persons of reproductive age) have not thus far materialized. Group violence, group suicide, flight or exodus, and the "final solution" of pogrom or genocide are probably largely dependent on HIV prevalence levels within groups, and the size and political or social position of those groups. The long periods between seroconversion and expression of clinical symptoms may serve to delay violent coping strategies but may hasten attempts at quarantine. Isolation of seropositive persons as well as those with frank AIDS already is occurring in the eastern United States in two ways: negatively and positively. Negative isolation take place when everyone uses masks, gloves, and gowns to keep from touching a person with AIDS, or even only suspected of being seropositive. This kind of de facto isolation is happening daily in courtroom holding pens, jails, prisons and, in fact, wherever blood is or could be spilled, as at the scene of accidents or on school premises.[21] Positive isolation or quarantine of unlimited duration is being effected by the creation of housing, hospital wards, and hospices for those with AIDS.[22]

A possible effect of both negative and positive isolation may be violence against self or others. In the eastern United States the issue of suicide has become associated with the right to die in the context of terminal illness [see reference 4]. There are media reports and anecdotal accounts of suicide and attacks on others by AIDS patients in both the eastern United States and East Africa. One form of attack is the attempt to deliberately infect others by biting or, with prior knowledge of one's own seropositivity, by sexual intercourse.[23] In the eastern United States there are also reports of increased violence against homosexuals; it would seem a matter of time and prevalence levels before such attacks are directed against larger targets: government agencies, including the military, as well as against entire ethnic or racial groups.[24]

Finally, and in contrast to the violent and negative projection just made, there are the positive coping strategies of the World Health Organization and other national and international agencies at the scale of the largest groups of all, continental and hemispheric. The recognition and accumulation of information on HIV transmission at these levels is the best hope for the future.

Discussion

The two paradigms, one for size of group affected by AIDS and HIV infection, and the other for coping strategies, can only be related to each other in an ad hoc fashion. For these paradigms to become more internally coherent it will probably be necessary to recognize additional variables. This will require additional research both in the existing literature on the anthropology and sociology of the two regions, and in the field. Ideally, social scientists (especially those from the countries involved) who are expert in the regions being investigated should participate at every stage of epidemiological investigation, from original protocol design (to ensure that questions are asked in culturally acceptable eliciting frames), to fieldwork (to ensure that sampling design and procedures are followed), to interpretation of the results. The participation of social scientists can also help to avoid pejorative labeling. Too often the social scientist is brought in too late to solve problems originally caused by cultural insensitivity, poor questionnaire design, and unfamiliarity with regional interconnections. In fact, in my experience, there can be a real confusion in the minds of those in the biomedical and health professions between social science and social work. It is as though the "science" of social science could be done by anyone with training in science of whatever kind. But the *work* of social science, is not that "social work"? Largely at issue here is a failure to realize that sociocultural awareness (gained through intense involvement in the literature and fieldwork) is a resource needed at every level of hypothesis formulation, research planning, and execution. To date, however, few (if any) of the national committees cooperating with the World Health Organization include social scientists among their members.

Even at present and without such thorough integration of the social and biomedical disciplines as suggested above, it is possible to suggest additional factors affecting the choices a people will make for coping with the AIDS epidemic. One such factor is the sometimes very slow development from seroconversion to frank AIDS. Another factor affecting invoked strategies surely is relatable to the appearance and physical condition of the seropositive persons or those with clinical AIDS. Prolonged fever, weight loss, and diarrhea are so common in developing areas of the tropics that diagnosis of AIDS need not be definitive for the patient, neighbors, family, or kin—at least for a while. To the extent that ambiguity is preserved, some of the more acute or violent strategies for coping with the effects of HIV infection may be defused. In a region where symptoms of AIDS are quite distinctive from background health conditions, reactions to the disease may be quicker, and more pointed. Still another factor that may affect choice of strategy is the extent to which a government agency, whether it is a laboratory, a health department, a police force, or the military is perceived as a carrier of the virus. Such a perception, of course, might lead to open defiance and escalation of coping strategies to include flight and exodus, or worse.

None of the larger groups (regional, national, and continental) have become involved in concerted coping strategies. Nor have the most active or violent strategies been invoked. With fuller understanding of the social consequences of AIDS, they may never be. Should present coping strategies persist or become more violent, however, populations in both the East African and eastern United States regions may become accustomed to isolation, de facto quarantine, and violence against *all* those in prolonged ill health including those with AIDS. This psycho-cultural consequence, amounting to an insensitivity and even brutality toward those with prolonged illness, may be more tragic in the long run than the infectivity and morality rates now associated with HIV infection and AIDS.[25]

Conclusions

The East African region and the eastern United States are so different in so many ways that it is easy to be blinded to some important features and processes they have in common: both regions are complex in the sense of being culturally mixed and socially stratified; they contain mobile populations and migrant individuals; urban areas are expanding, and there are extensive "foreign" enclaves and multiple international connections. Great differences in physical environments, cultural history, and in many social institutions do not override these similarities, each of which is potentially significant in terms of viral transmission, the spread of AIDS, coping strategies, and the social consequences of these illnesses. The two paradigms presented here for discovering some of these regional similarities do not have predictive value. Their only value is heuristic.

On the basis of the foregoing, one conclusion is that there may be many more AIDS-related parallels in East Africa and the eastern United States than have been discussed here. A second conclusion is that each region may forecast for the other some of the social consequences of AIDS. A third conclusion is that the perception of parallels between otherwise contrastive regions is heightened by the use of paradigms or scalar representations of common cultural, sociological, and epidemiological factors. Further research may enhance the development of useful paradigms to the point where they do become predictive. This will require integration of the health and social sciences, however, to a degree not yet achieved. Finally, tragic as the personal and demographic consequences of AIDS may be at present, the social consequences could become worse. Better integrated research may help avoid them by enabling us to identify and implement alternative and more humane coping strategies.

References and Notes

1. P. Piot, F.A. Plummer, F.S. Mhalu, J-L. Lamboray, J. Chin, J.M. Mann, *Science* **239**, 573 (1988). In the references that follow, *The New York Times* is abbreviated as *NYT*. A letter preceding a page number indicates the section of the edition for that date. For international travel and AIDS screening for aliens in the United States and Russia, see *NYT*, A1, 9 June 1987; 22, 19 July 1987; B4, 21 July 1987; B5, 27 Aug. 1987; 8, 29 Aug. 1987; A11, 17 Sept. 1987. For additional international dimensions of AIDS see L.C. Chen, *Daedalus*, **116**, 181 (1987). References to the social consequences of AIDS are being collected and maintained in a database for microcomputers at the Human Ecology and Remote Sensing Laboratory in the Department of Anthropology at Hunter College, NY. Inquiries are welcome.

2. For resort to alternative health care in the eastern United States see *NYT* A21, 16 March 1988; C3, 15 March 1988. See also the *AIDS/ARC News List*, and *AIDS/ARC Treatment News* available via BITNET AIDSNEWS@RUTVM1. For African alternative health care systems prior to AIDS, see J.M. Janzen, *The Quest for Therapy: Medical Pluralism in Lower Zaire* (Indiana Univ. Press, Bloomington, 1978) and Z.A. Ademuwagu, J. Ayoade, I. Harrison, D. Warren, Eds., *African Therapeutic Systems* (Crossroads Press, Los Angeles, 1979).

3. On the hospice solution, see *NYT*, B1, 12 June 1987; B1, 12 June 1987; B1, 55, 22 Sept. 1987.

4. On AIDS suicide and right-to-die, see *NYT*, B3, 16 July 1987; B18, 28 July 1987; 6, 4 Oct. 1987.

5. For the early years of AIDS see R. Shilts, *And the Band Played On* pp. 234–252 (St. Martin's Press, New York). For reluctance in East Africa to confront AIDS see C. Norman, *Science* **230**, 1140 (1985), D. Dickson, *Science* **238**, 605 (1987). See also *NYT*, 23, 8 Feb. 1987; A2, 29 May 1987. For subsequent changes in policy, see *NYT*, 25, 1 Nov. 1987; A8, 5 Oct. 1987; A1, 8 Feb. 1987; A11, 19 Feb. 1988.

6. For the economic plight of women in accessing AIDS assistance in the eastern United States see *NYT*, 1, 6 March 1988; A1, 27 Aug. 1987; A18, 30 Sept. 1987.

7. For only two recommendations for sexual abstinence, see *NYT*, B7, 7 Oct. 1987 (Education Secretary Bennett) and *NYT* A1, 8 June 1987 (New York City, Mayor Koch).

8. For Nairobi prostitutes from the epidemiological point of view see J.K. Kreiss, *et al.*, *The N. Engl. J. Med.* **314**, 414 (1986). For the use of "free woman" as equivalent of "prostitute" see N. Nzilambi *et al.*, *The N. Engl. J. Med.* **318**, 276 (1988).

9. For a detailed socio-historical account of women in Nairobi, see L. Whyte, *Signs* **11**, 255 (1986).

10. See *NYT* A17, 5 June 1987. See also *NYT* A14, 27 March 1987; B1, 7 January 1988; and *US News & World Report* (16 Feb. 1987) for "class" prostitutes in Nevada and Japan.

11. See, for example, *NYT*, C18, 24 Sept. 1987 for the resettlement of the Ray children in Florida.

12. For difficulty in maintaining AIDS-affected children in school see *NYT* B4, 24 Dec. 1987.
13. For public policy with respect to "pediatric AIDS" see The Citizen's Committee for Children of New York, *The Invisible Emergency: Children and AIDS in New York* (The Committee, 105 E. 22 St., New York 10010, 1987); *Surgeon General's Workshop on Children with HIV Infection and their Families*, (Division of Maternal and Child Health, Rockville, MD, 1987). See also *NYT*, B8, 9 Apr. 1987; A21, 14 Dec. 1987. On nurseries in hospitals, see *NYT*, B4, 17 July 1987; B1, 8 May 1987. On fostering and foster homes see *NYT*, B18, 28 July 1987; 69, 13 Sept. 1987.
14. On difficulties of providing AIDS care by family members, see B. Peabody, *The Screaming Room: A Mother's Journal of Her Son's Struggle with AIDS*. (Oak Tree Publishers, San Francisco, 1986). For family coping, see also *NYT Magazine* (21 June 1987) and *US News and World Report*, (12 Oct. 1987). For difficulty in eastern United States in AIDS persons leaving the city and returning to the countryside, see *NYT*, A1, 2 Nov. 1987; B1, 17 Nov. 1986.
15. On the effect of AIDS on age cohorts, see especially the work of J. Bongaarts, Institute of Medicine, *Approaches to Modeling Disease Spread and Impact: Report of a Workshop on Mathematical Models of the Spread of Human Immunodeficiency Virus and the Demographic Impact of Acquired Immunodeficiency Syndrome* (National Academy Press, Washington, DC, 1988). On the resiliency of African systems for recruitment and replacement, see G. Merritt, Workshop on Cultural Factors in AIDS Overseas, AAAS Annual Meeting, 11 February 1988.
16. For eastern United States, New York City has been mapped for varying rates of AIDS prevalence. See *NYT*, 1, 13 Dec. 1987. For difficulty in reaching Black and Hispanic inner-city residents, see R. Goldstein, *The Village Voice*, (10 March 1987).
17. Some ethnic and inner-city information is provided on Kinshasa by J.M. Mann, *et al., J. Am. Med. Assoc.* **255**, 3255 (1986). Research and news coverage on rural areas is thin. See Nzilambi (*8*) for a rural area in Zaire. The Uganda village of Kyebe has perhaps received the most intense news coverage. See *NYT*, C1, 30 Sept. 1986.
18. For government reluctance in the eastern United States towards developing AIDS policy see W. Booth, *Science*, **838**, 237 (1987); *NYT*, A1, 10 Aug. 1987. For positive reaction to changes in policy, see *NYT*, A32, 21 Feb. 1988. See also Shilts in Note 5.
19. For examples of the use of Haiti as a label see *NYT*, 1, 29 June 1986; A8, 28 July 1986. See J. Mann, *New Scientist*, 40 (26 March 1987) for earlier reactions in Africa to "finger pointing" and assumptions about sexual habits.
20. For continuing delay in releasing AIDS information relating to laboratory workers, see *NYT*, 37, 1 Jan. 1988.
21. On negative isolation and the use of "protective" clothing for court room personnel, see *NYT*, 55, 16 Aug. 1987; A12, 22 June 87. Media reports on the use of special clothing for fire fighters, police, and hospital workers are too numerous to be included here. For the distribution of gloves to New York City schoolteachers, see *NYT*, 1, 10 Oct. 1987.
22. On positive isolation in hospital wards and hospices, see *NYT* A15, 27 Jan. 1988; A12, 2 Jan. 1987; A21, 2 Dec. 1987; 30, 13 June 1987; B9, 17 June 1987.

23. For examples of accusations of deliberate HIV transmission by United States military personnel, see *NYT,* A25, 3 Mar. 1988; B5, 4 Dec. 1987; A5, 17 Nov. 1987; 4, 21 Feb. 1987; 31, 4 Apr. 1987; B9, 8 May 1987. On public reactions in Bavaria, see *NYT,* Section 4, 30, 12 July 1987. For accusations of deliberate transmission by a male prostitute, see *NYT* B4, 13 Feb. 1987. For biting, see *NYT,* B3, 3 Sept. 1987 (Connecticut); A29, 10 June 1987 (Manhattan); A18, 25 June 1987 (Minneapolis); 11, 7 June 1987 (Brazil).

24. On AIDS as an inducement to bank robbery, see *NYT* B3, 25 Aug. 1987. On violence against the AIDS affected, see NYT B4, 26 August 1987, on bomb threats against the Florida school accepting the Ray brothers [see Note 11]. For attacks on homosexuals, see *NYT,* A12, 24 Apr. 1987. For reactions involving the military, see *NYT,* B4, 24 Feb. 1987 (Kenya); A1, 27 Dec. 1986 (Philippines); on the military and civilians, see *NYT,* A20, 23 April 1987; A13, 24 April 1987; B4, 2 Sept. 1987. For civil protest (California) over the cost of AIDS medication, see *NYT,* D23, 9 Feb. 1988.

25. Encouragement and criticism by colleagues, including R. Berk, D. Bates, and V. Redi, as well as the research assistance of Y. Gabre-Medhin, A. Mathews, E. Milman, and K. Morrell are gratefully acknowledged. The research has been supported in part by funding from the CUNY-PSC awards program.

About the Authors

Paul Abramson is an Associate Professor of Psychology at the University of California, Los Angeles and current editor of *The Journal of Sex Research*.

Richard A. Berk is a Professor of Sociology and Social Statistics at the University of California, Los Angeles. He is Vice-Chairperson of the Social Sciences Research Council Board of Directors and Chair of the Methodology Section of the American Sociological Association.

Francis Conant is on the faculty of the Anthropology Department at Hunter College, City University of New York. He is also Director of the Human Ecology and Remote Sensing Laboratory there.

Christopher Corey is a graduate student and research assistant in the Department of Sociology at the University of California, Los Angeles. He has co-authored a number of papers with Drs. Freeman and Lewis on access to health services and primary care physicians' AIDS-related knowledge and behaviors.

Howard E. Freeman is Professor and Chair of the Department of Sociology at the University of California, Los Angeles, where he formerly was Director of the Institute for Social Science Research.

Alice Horrigan is a journalist and graduate student of sociology at the University of California, Los Angeles. She studied liberation theology in Nicaragua, Peru, and Brazil as a fellow of the Thomas J. Watson Foundation during 1982–1983.

James Kinsella, editor of editorial pages at the Los Angeles Herald Examiner, was a fellow at Columbia University's Gannett Center during 1987–1988. His book on media coverage of AIDS is forthcoming in the fall of 1989.

Charles Lewis is Chief of the Division of General Internal Medicine, Department of Medicine, at the University of California, Los Angeles. He is currently undertaking and evaluating innovative community-based AIDS-prevention programs in Los Angeles.

Robin Lloyd is a Ph.D. candidate in Sociology at the University of California, Santa Barbara. She is interested in social responses to AIDS, conversation in institutional settings, gender, and medical sociology; her current work analyzes radio conversations between paramedics and nurses.

Beth E. Schneider is an Associate Professor of Sociology at the University of California, Santa Barbara. She is currently a member of the Sex/Gender Council (ASA), the Santa Barbara County AIDS Planning Council, and the Sociologists' AIDS Network.

Bernard Weiner is a Professor of Psychology at the University of California, Los Angeles. His major research concerns are in the areas of motivation and emotion, from an attributional perspective.

Other Abt Books about AIDS

The Heterosexual Transmission of AIDS in Africa
Dieter Koch-Weser, M.D., Ph.D. and Hannelore Vanderschmidt, Ph.D., editors

This unique source book comprises sixty-two scientific articles from *The Lancet, Science, Annales Institut Pasteur* and other journals and describes the scope and intensity of the AIDS epidemic in Africa. Topics include the origins of AIDS; the discovery of HIV2 in West Africa; African epidemiology, serology, and virology; the relationship of heterosexual transmission to prostitution and promiscuity; the relationship of AIDS to other diseases; and the differences between the transmission of AIDS in Africa and in the United States. **1988.**

Cloth: ISBN 0-89011-603-2   *Paper: ISBN 0-89011-604-0*

AIDS and Law Enforcement
Theodore M. Hammett, Ph.D. and Dana Hunt, Ph.D., editors

A comprehensive and thoughtful look at how AIDS affects the law enforcement and criminal justice systems. The authors examine training and education for law enforcement staff and offenders; use of law enforcement officers as AIDS educators in the community; pros and cons of HIV antibody testing, and alternatives to testing; housing decisions; precautionary measures; confidentiality and notification issues; emerging legal issues and case law; and the development of a rational and responsible justice system. **1989.**

Cloth: ISBN 0-89011-605-9   *Paper: ISBN 0-89011-606-7*

AIDS and HIV Antibody Testing: Pros and Cons
Theodore M. Hammett, Ph.D. and Dana Hunt, Ph.D., editors

A collection of recent papers by distinguished social scientists, giving both sides of the testing argument. An original introduction by Drs. Theodore Hammett and Dana Hunt describes currently available tests, looks at the meaning of test results, and discusses prospects for improved testing technology. The contributors evaluate the purposes of testing, and discuss related issues of accuracy, reliability, confidentiality, and counseling. They also examine the implications of testing for blood supply, military recruitment, employment, prison and corrections staff populations, immigration, hospital admissions, and marriage licensing. **1989.**

Cloth: ISBN 0-90011-607-5   *Paper: ISBN 0-89011-608-3*

All titles are available from Abt Books, 146 Mount Auburn Street, Cambridge, Massachusetts 02138.